Reforming Child Protection

**Bob Lonne, Nigel Parton,
Jane Thomson and
Maria Harries**

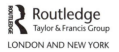 Routledge
Taylor & Francis Group

LONDON AND NEW YORK

First published 2009
by Routledge
2 Park Square, Milton Park, Abingdon, Oxon OX14 4RN

Simultaneously published in the USA and Canada
by Routledge
270 Madison Avenue, New York, NY 10016

*Routledge is an imprint of the Taylor & Francis Group,
an informa business*

© 2009 Bob Lonne, Nigel Parton, Jane Thomson and Maria Harries

Typeset in Times New Roman by
Florence Production Ltd, Stoodleigh, Devon
Printed and bound in Great Britain by
CPI Antony Rowe, Chippenham, Wiltshire

British Library Cataloguing in Publication Data
A catalogue record for this book is available from the British Library

Library of Congress Cataloging in Publication Data
Reforming child protection/Bob Lonne . . . [*et al.*].
    p. cm.
  1. Child welfare – English-speaking countries.
  2. Children – Services for – English-speaking countries.
  3. Social work with children – English-speaking countries.
  I. Lonne, Bob.
HV713.R44 2008
362.7–dc22   2007052724

ISBN10: 0–415–42905–6 (hbk)
ISBN10: 0–415–42906–4 (pbk)
ISBN10: 0–203–89467–7 (ebk)

ISBN13: 978–0–415–42905–4 (hbk)
ISBN13: 978–0–415–42906–1 (pbk)
ISBN13: 978–0–203–89467–5 (ebk)

This book is dedicated to those who supported us throughout the process of planning and writing it—our partners, children and grandchildren.

It is also dedicated to the many people who, like us, are passionate advocates for children and families, and believe that things can be done better than they are at present. Reform processes are never easy. Keep the passion!

Contents

Illustrations

Figures

Tables

Foreword

Bob Lonne, Nigel Parton, Jane Thomson, and Maria Harries have written an *important* book—a descriptor that I rarely apply. In regard, however, to *Reforming Child Protection*, the attribution is apt.

Broadly speaking, my assessment of the significance of Lonne *et al.*'s work is based on four factors. First, the authors effectively *challenge the conventional wisdom* about the necessary elements in the assurance of children's safety in their homes. Describing a system that is long on blame and short on helpfulness, Lonne *et al.* copiously document the bankruptcy of the prevailing child protection system in the English-speaking industrialized countries of Oceania, North America, and Europe.

Although Lonne *et al.* do not make this point, the central features of what they describe as the "Anglophone" approach to child protection are unfortunately being emulated by the many new democracies—regardless of their linguistic culture—that look to the United States and the United Kingdom for model policies (see, e.g., Lewis *et al.*, 2004; see also Mathews and Kenny, 2008, listing countries that generally follow the Anglophone model in their legislative framework for child protection). Further, the Anglophone approach is arguably embedded in the letter—but not the spirit—of international human rights law (Convention on the Rights of the Child, 1989, art. 19, § 2, requiring the development of a system of "identification, reporting, referral, [and] investigation" of suspected child abuse and neglect, language that originated primarily on motion of the representative of the United States; see Office of the United Nations High Commissioner for Human Rights, 2007). Hence, Lonne *et al.*'s criticisms potentially have global significance.

Second, Lonne *et al.* demonstrate a remarkable *ethical sensitivity*—in effect, a psychological-mindedness—in describing both the problems of the current system and the possibilities for a new one. They give due deference to the concerns of parents and children, they show similar respect for family (and family-like) relationships, and they avoid the common but ethically troublesome practice of arrogantly presuming that their own view of children's "best interests" trumps all relevant value judgments.

The importance of this perspective, which many readers might believe would be self-evident, is that it so vividly contrasts with much of prevailing practice. Too often, legal fictions overcome children's own experience. For example, children are assumed either to be in their parents' care or in substitute care; the reality that there is a continuum of supplementary care (most of which is well short of a full substitution) is ignored. Similarly, if children are placed in foster care, it is assumed that the only options are "reunification" or "adoption"; the overarching value on "permanence" disregards the reality of ambivalent but nonetheless important relationships. The assumption that there is severe harm as a result of even fleeting exploitation or abuse—no matter whether there is evidence of such *harm*—ignores the central question of whether a child has been *wronged*.

Even more egregiously, the current child protection system objectifies the children whom it seeks to protect and the parents whom it accuses. The ostensible mission of the system is lost as children are treated as evidence and "treatments" are designed to provide verification of parents' failures. In effect, a culture of caring is replaced by a culture of surveillance.

Lonne *et al.* recognize that this problem cannot be solved by merely increasing resources, efficiency, or accountability. They properly bemoan the preemption of "relationship-based social work" by "case-management-driven proceduralism" and the corollary loss of both meaning and respect in workers' interaction with children and parents.

Third, the fact that the authors are luminaries in the social work profession on two continents brings a *special credibility* to observations and opinions that might otherwise be rejected out of hand. A common problem of reform in child protection is that efforts to relieve social service providers from inherently unrealistic expectations have often been misinterpreted by professional guilds as attacks on the specialty child protection division of social service agencies—Child Protective Services—and the social work profession.

I observed such defensiveness when the US Advisory Board on Child Abuse and Neglect (1991), of which I was then vice-chair, made its initial effort to bring other professions and agencies into active participation in the child protection system:

> The Board members shared strong beliefs that, to be effective, child protection must become part of everyday life and that, to accomplish such a goal, it must be comprehensive—built into the fabric of every community institution. Such an approach implies the need to reduce not only the burden but also the centrality of the specialty child welfare system in the protection of children. Child protection is not simply or even primarily a job for social service agencies.
>
> At the time, this conclusion was actively resisted by the Washington-based organizations that represent public child welfare agencies and their staff or that have historically been closely allied with them. Thus, recommendations that might have been expected to be uncontroversial were perceived as threatening by groups that perceived a diminution of their role in child protection.

(Melton, 2002: 573)

Such resistance is ironic. Efforts to build a comprehensive child protection system potentially liberate service providers from inherently unrealistic expectations. Moreover, the values and strategies that Lonne *et al.* and other reformers are attempting to bring to the forefront are those that historically have been associated with social work. In short, the approach that is being advocated is one that supports the best traditions of the profession.

Fourth, even if one perceives the changes that Lonne *et al.* advocate as somehow radical, they are *achievable*. As Lonne *et al.* note, the greatest achievement of the child protection system in the second half of the twentieth century was that "it is now an exception rather than a rule to have adults who do not recognize the significance and scope of child abuse and neglect, and who support the obligation of the broad community to intervene to protect vulnerable children." Building from this concern, it is time to use the collective sense of responsibility to build or strengthen universal systems of support for families.

I am currently leading Strong Communities for Children, a long-term, foundation-sponsored initiative to implement the US Advisory Board's (1993b) vision in parts of two counties in northwestern South Carolina (see Melton and Holaday, 2008). In an ethnically diverse, mixed-social-class area with rural, small-town, suburban, and urban communities (approximately 125,000 people, according to the 2000 census), we have sought to prevent child maltreatment by strengthening the ties among neighbors. Specifically, we have sought to assure that "no families are left outside," indeed that all children and parents in our service area will know that whenever they have reason to celebrate, worry, or grieve, someone will notice, and someone will care.

To do so, we have relied on hundreds of community organizations, especially those in primary institutions (religious organizations, fire departments, community police officers, primary health clinics, civic clubs, and others) that are rarely perceived as key elements of child protection. In this context, in less than 6 years, we have engaged almost 5,000 volunteers who have contributed more than 50,000 hours (a conservative estimate). Moreover, we have been most successful in the least advantaged communities.

In an era of alienation and isolation, we have shown that it is still feasible to bring people together to weave safety nets for children and their families. I mention Strong Communities, because we have generated such support in an area that is among the most conservative in the United States, both politically and theologically. Upstate South Carolina would not be predicted by most observers to be fertile ground for an initiative to enhance child welfare, even if primarily through informal support in the community. Nonetheless, the desire to "Keep Kids Safe"—to ensure the security of the smallest members of the community—transcends ideology; moreover, it overpowers the social differences that often divide communities.

As I write this foreword in January 2008, I am watching television coverage of the results of the South Carolina Democratic primary, an election won with a landslide by Barack Obama. In both parties, the theme of the current election is the need for *change*—in particular, change directed toward bringing people together, regardless of their ideology, wealth, ethnicity, religion, or politics.

Although this theme undoubtedly reflects in part the enormous unpopularity of the Bush presidency, both domestically and internationally, I suspect that the belief that it is time to bring people together reflects a hunger that is much deeper and broader. For at least a generation, strong centrifugal forces have pushed people—especially young adults (therefore, most of the parents of young children)—further and further apart, all the way across the industrialized world (Pharr and Putnam, 2000). In such an era of disconnection and distrust, parents perceive that the community available to support their children and to assist parents themselves in their care for their children is ever thinner. In that context, people find it ever easier to imagine circumstances in which otherwise good parents can have lapses in their supervision and nurturance of their children, especially when poverty, illness, or environmental danger make those tasks more difficult.

When the US Advisory Board was debating the feasibility of a neighborhood-based strategy for child protection in discussions that often went far into the night, I was most moved by a member's account of a colleague's plaintive revelation that he felt locked in a war for the hearts and minds of his children. My own pride in the social concern and personal resilience of my young adult daughters is accompanied by worry that they may lack the web of support that sustained the generations before them.

Although community has a special meaning in American culture (Toqueville, 1835/2000), and its loss therefore has especially great significance in my country (Putnam 2000), the sense that it is time to strengthen ties among people in general—and especially among parents—is one that can be felt across the globe (Melton, 1993). It is time for change! *Reforming Child Protection* is an important step in building the intellectual foundation for such transformation, at least in the systems directly responsible for the well-being of the most vulnerable children.

Gary B. Melton
Institute on Family and Neighborhood Life
Clemson University
Clemson, South Carolina, USA

Abbreviations

ABCAN	US Advisory Board on Child Abuse and Neglect
ARC	availability, responsiveness and continuity
CAF	Common Assessment Framework
CALD	culturally and linguistically diverse
CAPTA	Child Abuse and Prevention and Treatment Act
CCR	child concern report
CMA	child maltreatment allegation
CMC	Crime and Misconduct Commission
EBP	evidence-based practice
HREOC	Human Rights and Equal Opportunities Commission
HRM	human resource management
ICS	Integrated Children's System
ICT	information and communication technology
IS Index	Information Sharing Index
NGO	non-government organization
NPM	New Public Management
NSPCC	National Society for the Prevention of Cruelty to Children
SPCC	Society for the Prevention of Cruelty to Children
TSA	US Transportation Security Administration
UNCROC	United Nations Convention on the Rights of the Child

Part I

Reforming child protection

Introduction: an overview

1 Reforming child protection

Principles and themes of effective child, family, and community well-being

In this chapter we introduce our central thesis and provide an outline of the core principles that inform it. Fundamental to our analysis is the reality of the now well recognized systemic failure of the child protection systems that operate in Anglophone countries and their underlying paradigm. We describe the elements of this paradigm and outline in some detail how an alternative and effective system of child well-being could work to support children, parents, families, and communities, as well as providing a safe haven for children for whom care within their birth family is no longer possible. We also recognize that this is a work in progress and that there is further effort to be done in fleshing out the conceptual framework so that it can be operationalized in the day-to-day practice of service providers. The first half of the book consists of a critique of contemporary Anglophone child protection systems and practice. In the second half we propose a new framework and explain the components of this. Values are at the core of each of the elements of the comprehensive model that we put forward.

It is important to clarify at the outset what we mean by Anglophone countries and to note that, while they share some common features, there are indeed significant jurisdictional variations between them. The countries to which we refer are the United States of America, Canada, the United Kingdom, Australia, and New Zealand. These countries are united in their approaches to the care and protection of children in the following ways:

- They tend to use the term "child protection" services.
- Most of them are highly forensic and focused primarily on assessment of risk to children by family or caregivers.
- Services tend to be extremely managerialized structures and processes with priority given to risk-averse practices and highly legalized procedures.
- The referral portal tends to be one in which reports and referrals are for "children at risk" rather than "child or family in need."
- Most of them have mandatory reporting legislation (or its equivalent such as reporting protocols) that requires the reporting to a statutory authority of any concern about harms or risks to children.

- Prevention and family support are generally accepted in the policies of the statutory authority for child protection, but are secondary to the primary role of child protection.

While acknowledging these similarities, it is also important to note that what is implicit in the descriptors above is that there are idiosyncrasies between the jurisdictions. Some of these will become clear in the book. One of the most significant differences sits on the continuum of forensic investigation and prevention. Most of these countries are highly forensically charged in their approach. In other words, once a child protection report or referral is made, the preoccupation and major tasks of the investigating person or team are:

- to assess whether harm has been done to a child or there is a risk of such harm (substantiate or support the allegation);
- to make a decision about whether or not to remove the child and charge parents or guardians; and
- to record the event on some form of register.

The situation in England and also in Scotland, Wales and Northern Ireland—though the detail is rather varied in each jurisdiction—is somewhat different. In recent years England has embarked on a major period of reform and change. In particular, the idea of child protection is now located in a much wider strategy of trying to "safeguard and promote the welfare of the child" (Parton 2006a,b) and the focus of assessment is the "child's needs" rather than risk. The last 10 years have witnessed considerable efforts at both the policy and practice levels to "refocus" children's services and to maximize the opportunities for all children particularly those who are the most deprived. We discuss the nature and implications of these developments throughout the book, particularly in Chapters 1 and 2. What we note is that while considerable change has taken place, the managerialist and proceduralized nature of the work has increased even further.

All four authors are social work trained and have a collective experience of child welfare spanning over 60 years. All of us work in Anglophone countries. We are also academics who teach in and research about child and family welfare, in three different universities in Australia, and in the United Kingdom. All four of us have been heavily involved in critically assessing and analyzing contemporary practices, and re-formulating policies and improving on-site training in order to generate practices that provide evidence of outcomes that really do protect and ensure the safety of highly vulnerable children, assist parents and families, and build communities. Our professional experience spans practice, policy, research, and management in government, non-government, and community services for vulnerable children, families, and communities. We have used our collective experience and research to inform this critical analysis of dominant contemporary approaches to what are generally called "child protection" services in these Anglophone countries.

Much has now been written about the universal systemic failures of child protection and welfare services—but particularly in the Anglophone world (Waldfogel 1998; Berg and Kelly 2000; Wharf 2002). Schorr (1998) suggests that the need for major reform of the child welfare system was already evident in the mid 1980s. By late 2007 as we complete this book, the expressed need for change is manifest—the crisis is evidenced in numerous publications, reports and public statements (Barter 2002; Melton *et al.* 2002; Melton 2005; Freymond and Cameron 2006; D. Scott 2006a; Mansell 2006a,b; Pelton 2008). There have always been the critics who have uttered warnings about the high likelihood of negative sequelae produced by an uncritical acceptance of the child rescue movement and the "child protection" imperatives. However, recently, the call for reform has been escalating with a number of scholars and practitioners from a range of disciplines telling us that the system is close to bankrupt (Melton 2005; Testro and Peltola 2007); that it may well be doing more harm than good (Swift 1997; D. Scott 2006a); that it is shattering families (Roberts 2002; Reich 2005) and communities with dire consequences for civil society (Smith 2005; Watson and Moran 2005; Webb 2006).

In the following chapters we describe the multifaceted aspects of contemporary child protection debates and argue that most of them are operating within a paradigm that has failed, despite its central tenet of protecting children and enhancing their well-being. We present compelling evidence from Anglophone countries that their child protection systems are haemorrhaging, and we make a case for a different approach, and propose a means for implementing it. Our primary aim in writing this book is to challenge the dominant paradigm in child protection that, we argue, has led to a significant dissonance between the aims and the outcomes of policies, and between the experiences of those who develop these policies and those who are the recipients of them.

It is indisputable that the term "child abuse" is a social and legal construct that emerged only in the 1960s and 1970s and became all-encompassing of a range of behaviors and attributes in the 1980s. Since then, the construct has taken on the very erroneous image of "having achieved universal consensus about what it constitutes" (Hoyano and Keenan 2007: 7) and, to use Ferguson's terms, has emerged "as a global idea and ideal" with a "powerful hold" in the Western world that is hard to challenge, despite its failures (Ferguson 2004: 3). The construct has also suffered from relentless definitional inflation (Thorpe 1997) and reporting data from across the Anglophone world have become almost meaningless as ever increasing "indicators" of abuse (such as emotional harm and obesity) are added to the endless lists attached to reporting requirements, and thereby contribute to the stark reality of child welfare systems that are in chaos and confusion.

While recognizing that there is a crisis in child protection/welfare services, we add that this crisis is also being documented in a number of human service areas. Examples of these are mental health, education, and prison (corrective) services where "new paradigms" are challenging policy makers and practitioners to fundamentally re-conceptualize the premises on which assessments are conducted, decisions are made and policies formulated (Read *et al.* 2004). There are lessons to be learned, in particular, from the quite dramatic worldwide changes in disability and mental health practices that have accompanied what is called "the consumer/carer movement" in which new hope has emerged for truly collaborative partnerships based on the acceptance of the wisdom and expertise that sits with the people who experience the problems that we are attempting to resolve, rather than simply with the "experts."

Pivotal to some of these changes is the notion that the priority competency for anyone working in mental health services, for example, is the capacity to understand the lived experience of the person with the mental illness and her/ his family, and the acceptance of the fact that respect is essential for the development of any working relationship that is the basis for positive outcomes for people. These changes in mental health, in particular, follow the discovery that appalling outcomes for people with disabilities or for those being treated for mental health problems have been highly correlated with the professionally driven deficit-model of traditional medical and psychiatric services (albeit that these are and have been established and driven by well-intentioned people).

It is perhaps unsurprising that services for vulnerable children and families have been slower than some other areas in the uptake of a new service paradigm despite the crescendo of demands for change. Perhaps this is because of the images of abused children, abusive parents and neglectful "bad mothers" which are imprinted in the community psyche and leave little room for movements that are interpreted as jeopardizing the lives of children. These powerful portrayals may well make it harder to change the paradigm for services aimed at safeguarding children from harm. Perhaps, as is suggested by some authors, child protection is a new industry intent on protecting its fledgling status and authority and, as such, cannot yet embrace a challenge to some of the fundamental premises that provide the very scaffolding for its existence. Or perhaps, the reasons are far more ordinary, and alternative ways of working have not been sufficiently well documented and researched and are not yet sufficiently convincing to enable change to occur. Some of this will become clearer as we explore in this book the issues of ethical practice, risk, and vulnerability, and power, and powerlessness—concepts that go to the very heart of professional interventions that seek to protect the vulnerable and alter the ways people behave.

In this book a number of premises are identified and critically examined. These include: the centrality of the need to care for and nurture children in every society; the endemic nature of structural problems among children considered to be at risk, as well as their families, neighborhoods, and communities; the profound effect of managerialism upon the practices of social care professionals in increasingly procedurally driven organizations; the stress on workers who have to manage competing professional and political agendas within an environment of fear; the iatrogenesis produced by risk-aversive practices; the power and politics of child protection discourses, and the identified failure of the current paradigm that is informing many Anglophone models of child protection. We then address the key challenges as we see them. These include:

- the need for a renewed focus on child and family well-being rather than investigation and surveillance;
- a new ethical framework with a well-articulated value base;
- a return to relationship-based practice and genuine partnerships with children and parents;
- professional and public health approaches that accept and manage risk;
- a renewed emphasis on the importance of working locally and assisting families;
- accessible and integrated programs and services that are embedded within neighborhoods and communities;
- engagement between practice-informed management and front-line staff;
- child- and family-informed practice; and
- a long-term focus on outcomes of children, families, neighborhoods and communities "over time."

In undertaking this analysis and critique, we honor the dedication and commitment of the many compassionate people who have worked hard over many years to draw attention to the needs of vulnerable children, and to protect them from abuse and harm: it is the paradigm that is in question, not the people. We propose far-reaching alternative approaches to the mechanisms for protecting and caring for children that recognize the complexity, fluidity and ambiguity of the work practitioners try to do. Our primary goal is to capitalize on opportunities to think differently about child safety in order to facilitate positive changes for children, families and communities—focusing on child and family well-being.

There are a number of key points that we make at the outset which serve to highlight and integrate the conceptualizations provided in each chapter. These ideas build on observations made by a number of contemporary scholars who have described recent developments in child protection in terms of moral panics generated by well-meaning people, and picked up by an eager media and an anxious public (Thomas 2002; Munro 1999b; Parton 1996; Waldfogel 1998; Callahan *et al.* (eds) 2000; Melton and Thompson 2002; Ainsworth and Hanson 2006). We contend that understandable moral panic has produced knee-jerk responses on the part of governments who want to be seen as "doing something" (Cohen 2002). They have done this in an evidential vacuum about what policies and practices work in different situations and environments (Wells 2006) opting instead, in many but not all jurisdictions, for a "one size fits all" forensic approach that is now acknowledged to be potentially harming as many people as it might help, and often not assisting those who are indeed harmed (Houston and Griffiths 2000; Pinkerton 2002; Mansell 2006a,b; D. Scott 2006a). What have emerged from the social angst and the panic are systems of risk-averse child protection, many of which are driven by pseudoscientific risk-assessment models and a preoccupation with procedures, rather than meaningful and practical assistance (Thomas 2002; Barter 2002).

We argue that the current narrow theoretical discourse of child protection is largely failing children and young people, and has embraced a commitment to technocratic risk assessment and a forensic approach to working with families. In pursuing this approach, professional judgment and the application of a combination of analytical and intuitive skills in working with people have been neglected as core practice imperatives. In essence, relationship-based social work has been supplanted by case management-driven proceduralism, which is devoid of meaningful and respectful engagement with children and parents, instead treating them as the "Other." The authors argue that the narrow child protection approach is part of the problem as to why we continue to experience record rates of maltreatment reports, unsubstantiated investigations and substantiated child harm, and why outcomes for children and young people who are alumni of the care system continue to be very poor. Therefore, while the authors will cover topics that other people in the field might expect to find, we will only include coverage of the current approaches across the globe in order to provide a critique of them, and propose an alternative approach.

As well as this, we contend that in the shadow of relentless child abuse inquiries, managerial systems are obsessed with the risk to themselves if they are perceived to be failing to protect children (Stanley and Manthorpe 2004). The solutions proposed to the problems we face in our policies and practices for protecting children generally follow on the heels of public scandals, child deaths and these subsequent inquiries. These solutions usually include developing or increasing a range of the following:

- reporting
- training
- risk assessment
- inter-agency collaboration.

So predictable are the recommendations to these inquiries that it led one commentator to observe that if we used similar methods to design an aircraft to that used to design our child protection systems, we would build such an aircraft only on the basis of analyzing the reasons for airplane crashes!

Generally, what follows an inquiry is that some system is found wanting; someone is found culpable either legally, administratively or morally; some suitable punishment (such as public admonishment, demotion or early retirement) follows; and the many invisible people who have had to continue working and providing care for children and families throughout the public conflagration continue their invisible, unrecognized but dedicated work. Alongside of all of this, reporting rates increase for a time; more reports are substantiated and more children are moved into the care system (Mansell 2006a,b); training programs (both professional and in-service) are developed (Barter 2002); risk assessment tools are revisited and tightened (Mansell 2006a,b); and agencies are called to develop new communication guidelines. All of these organizational redesigns occur in an environment of increased anxiety and risk for workers when, arguably, the preoccupation really needs to be on assisting workers to stay engaged and able to make complex assessments and judgments when working with the emotional heat that is generated in professional interventions with complex child and family problems.

The focus on risk assessment rather than beneficial service delivery outcomes is the hallmark of a large number of child protection systems that are no longer focused on proven outcomes and interventions such as the welfare and well-being of children or services to families. We argue that this preoccupation with developing and constantly refining risk assessment tools is aiding a course of failure. Current systems are over-focused on investigation and assessment rather than providing assistance, and are obsessed with the language of "risk," "perpetrators," and "offending parents"—all of which are alien to the lived experiences of most families who continue on with their lives in some form or other, regardless of the intervention that was aimed at investigation or assistance (Roberts 2002; Reich 2005). Children, young people and families often get help despite the system, not because of it, yet, many of the child protection systems that are in place actually militate against people referring themselves for assistance.

To add to these matters, we will argue that many child protection systems are punitive to everyone involved in them. Families who are subject to the unparalleled number of "unsubstantiated" reports are forgotten casualties of systems that focus on endless investigations in search of "perpetrators" (Harries and Clare 2002; D. Scott 2006a). Parents and children who are already vulnerable are often further damaged by overtly intrusive investigative procedures (Freymond and Cameron 2006; Family Inclusion Network 2007). Committed workers who have often dedicated long periods of their professional lives to improving the conditions for vulnerable children find themselves wounded by the relentlessness of the work, harried and hurt by uncompromising management-driven proceduralism, and burnt out and ostracized by a voracious media. Managers and politicians who are publicly pilloried because they don't have the solutions to what are generally deeply complex structural and contextual social problems, make ever more demands on workers in order to decrease the risk of agency liability and manage the pressures from a progressively more worried public.

Many of these systems are also inherently disrespectful about culture and other important differences. Legislation and policies that aim to address problems of child abuse generally assume a universal applicability that belies the inconsistencies within and between cultures, let alone between different regions and social groupings. In particular, Indigenous and Black children from minority populations and communities are grossly over-represented in child protection system reports, investigations, and interventions. In many ways this resembles neocolonization by dominant cultural groups (Fournier and Crey 1997; National Inquiry into the Separation of Aboriginal and Torres Strait Islander Children from their Families 1997; Roberts 2002).

Grounded in contemporary literature, research and scholarly inquiry, our book also capitalizes on recent research about the experiences and voices of children, young people, parents, and workers who are unarguably the most significant stakeholders in services pertaining to the care and protection of children. Indeed, it is in the voice of these key stakeholders that can be found some of the solutions to the way forward to really making a positive difference to the lives of children and families. The earlier paradigm that justifies any and all state intervention and paternalism in the name of adult-centric concerns for children is still overwhelmingly present today (Fox Harding 1996; Hill and Tisdall 1997). As the latter authors state so cogently "we still know far more about what adults think about children than we do directly from children themselves" (1997: 246), and this continues to be true despite the significant sociological research undertaken in recent years with children and young people (Parton 2006a). The problem of actually incorporating the wishes of children and young people becomes ever more fraught as we witness the rise of what is increasingly being termed our "risk society" with its concomitant reification of regulatory formulae for measurement and intervention— formulae that cannot afford to privilege the voice of the non-expert, that is the child, the youth or the parent (Webb 2006).

It needs to be acknowledged that the problem of incorporating the wishes of children and young people is also problematic when their role as agents assumes knowledge about the hugely complex domain of government activity and welfare health policy development. Parton (2006a) argues cogently that the very policies that are being developed in societies, such as in England, which aim to reduce secondary and tertiary intervention in the lives of children by developing primary prevention and public health approaches, are threatening to the rights of children and young people because they are all-pervasive. Most children and young people have no idea about the amount of information that is stored on files about them and, because they are generally not considered to be full citizens until they are 18 years old, they have no capacity to have any influence at this level. And, yet, it is interesting to contemplate the potential erosion of their rights when the state promotes a wholesale categorization of their lives from birth to adulthood—in the interests of their safety and well-being! How might this information be used during their childhood and, indeed, during their adulthood? For better or worse?

What has become more important, then, is not just finding out what children and young people think about but, rather, how they can influence adult lives and decision making—in particular, in this case, related to their safety and protection. Much of the current literature addresses the growing awareness of children as actors and agents rather than being simply objects of adult concern. We do know that children and young people want to be safe and we know that they want their families to be places where they can be safe. It would be a truism to say that most children and young people wish to remain with their family and to be safe. Indeed, most children who are harmed and neglected want foremost for this harm to stop and typically want their connection to, and relationship with, their parents and families to be reinforced and strengthened.

Our book is strongly values-based and presents an approach to practice that is best understood within a "virtue ethics" framework. That is, it establishes core values and principles for practice, recognizes the hugely complex and yet idiosyncratic family, neighborhood and community environments in which children and families struggle, and invites an inclusion of anticipated long- as well as short-term outcomes when decisions about the welfare of children are being made. It argues for a return to relationship and respect as core components of our work with children and families, and places this set of principles alongside the need to really understand and value culture, neighborhood and locality as the treasure chests for child safety and well-being.

It is important to recognize that the majority of the voices of opposition to much contemporary child protection practice such as ours, do not represent a countermovement to the need to care for and protect children that is suggested by authors such as Myers (1994) but, rather, they generally represent the concerns emerging from serious scholarship with families, communities, policy makers, and practitioners about what is working, and what is not working, and how we might care better for children. Our book does not argue against the centrality of the need to care for and protect the vulnerable: what it argues is that the methods that are being used are not meeting that need any more and, in many instances, are actually making situations worse for children. What we will argue throughout this book is that the predominance of an investigative/surveillance approach is largely excluding help being given. Or, to put it as provocatively as we do, "a preoccupation with social control is preventing the provision of social care."

In the USA where an escalating reporting, investigatory, and forensic child protection industry is now reported to be costing over $US100 billion annually and is recording over two million reports of child abuse or neglect per year, the child mortality rate from such abuse is increasing (Child Welfare Information Gateway 2006). In their recent fact sheet, this agency observes that there is an ongoing belief by US researchers that there continues to be an under-reporting of child abuse and mortality (2006: 2). In 1996 the UK Institute of Public Finance conservatively estimated the cost of child abuse to the country to be £1 billion a year. They comment:

> Most of this is spent dealing with the aftermath of abuse rather than its prevention. The total cost of abuse far exceeds this estimate. Individuals

and families bear most of the consequences, sometimes for the rest of their lives at an incalculable cost.

(NSPCC Inform 2004: 12)

In Australia, child abuse and neglect are estimated to cost taxpayers $5 billion each year and child protection authorities are reported to be overwhelmed with reporting numbers that have skyrocketed from 107,134 in 1999–2000 to 266,745 in 2005–06 (AIHW 2006). As disconcerting as are these data, is the low rate of what is called in Australia "substantiation of abuse" (as low as one fifth in many jurisdictions) and the absence of evidence that families and children who are reported are getting a service (D. Scott 2006a).

Neglect is the most common form of "maltreatment" in countries that have adopted screening and reporting mechanisms—40–60 percent (Shireman 2003; Watson 2004). Neglect is highly correlated with poverty, isolation, single parenthood, mental health and substance abuse. Many researchers have testified to the endemic nature of structural problems among children considered to be at risk of neglect (Thorpe 1994). Domestic violence, substance misuse and mental health problems are all reported as causative factors in the rising numbers of reports. There is little doubt that this has led to an overloaded system as we have also increasingly grafted on to child protection services the challenge of responding to domestic violence (Humphreys 2007). While acknowledging the importance of recognizing the impact of violence on children, Humphreys challenges the notion that child protection services have the capacity, let alone the appreciation or value base, that enable them to respond effectively, efficiently, efficaciously, or even ethically to the needs of children and families caught up in cycles of family violence that breed in disadvantaged communities.

It is interesting to note that as well as managing the now increased emotional stress, workers are also directed to increase their communications with workers in other agencies, and to do so with complicated new guidelines and inter-agency protocols. Yet the problem identified by inquiries has rarely been found to be lack of information. The problem is how this information is used and applied: it appears to often be about decision making—one of the toughest components of the work. A recent report commissioned by the Scottish Executive to investigate decision making in relation to two particular cases had this to say:

> It is hard to make sense of how so much professional energy could be devoted to sharing so much information, to such little effect, for the safety and welfare of the children in [this family]. Tough decisions to remove children were not taken quickly enough.
>
> (Scottish Executive 2005: 125)

It is, of course, evident that once the furore following the death or injury to a child is over and the media and public are reassured that the problem is solved—generally because more money and tighter controls have been promised—political interest in the care and protection of children plateaus or goes downwards. At this stage, while all else "returns to normal," front-line workers return to the unenviable task of providing services to children and families who are often suffering significant and sometimes chronic adversity. Staff typically counter this with an increased anxiety about the risk of imperfectly assessing the needs, problems, and capacities of families in service organizations that have few actual resources for helping to meet the needs of these children and families. And, for them, they are now even more clear that to do an imperfect assessment means facing the possibility of having to manage or survive management intervention, the media and public scrutiny, and shaming, and intense personal suffering that has pursued their professional colleagues during the media blitz. That this only happens relatively rarely is beside the point. The fear instilled in practitioners by the threat of it occurring has become a key component of organizational cultures and climates. We need not wonder why child welfare services experiences impossibly high turnover rates or why retention of any staff, let alone good staff, becomes the preoccupying concern of management of these agencies.

In contrast to the narrow child protection framework of which we are critical, this book claims a distinctive approach that is "cutting edge," in that it proposes a different and integrated theoretical paradigm for understanding the issues. The book has relevance for a broad readership, including practitioners, as their practice must be guided by theoretical underpinnings and the use of evidence in order for them to have a socially responsible mandate for intervention in the lives of vulnerable children and their families. Moreover, the value and ethical framework of much child protection practice often embraces overly punitive social control and a blaming approach that undermines the ability of families, neighborhoods and communities to provide nurturing and safe environments for children and young people. In this book, we propose a reinvigorated ethical framework to guide social work and welfare practice and the intervention of the state into family life. We argue that the contemporary environment leaves practitioners and managers with a potentially increased level of anxiety and uncertainty; and it leaves scholars and researchers trying to find answers to what is undoubtedly a crisis in service confidence in child protection services. What is needed is a theoretical and practice framework that articulates the links between values, theory, practice, evidence, and outcomes—for children and families.

In this book we aim to contribute to a common goal to build better solutions to the problem of protecting children and families experiencing adversity, and to help shape a new vision that enables us to keep children and families safe. Removal of children and young people from family and kin is justified when it is absolutely evident that the overall outcome is that it will actually protect them and enhance their long-term well-being, that is, their "well-being in time" (Ferguson 2004). To do this we add our challenge to that of others who have called for a new paradigm (Berg and Kelly 2000;

Houston and Griffiths 2000; Barter 2002; Testro and Peltola 2007) and we articulate some of the requirements for change.

The changes we recommend require policy makers, management, and practitioners to accept a challenge that requires them to:

- suspend belief in the way we are claiming to protect children in Anglophone countries;
- engage with an evidenced-based critique of the significant iatrogenic outcomes of contemporary Anglophone child protection practice;
- listen to children, parents, families, and communities;
- attend to alternative international approaches;
- pay attention to the voices of indigenous and minority peoples;
- review the ethical principles that should inform how we work with children and families;
- reinstate management arrangements that restore trust and respect for judgment to professional practitioners; and
- be honest with the public about the limits of our capacities to protect all children.

We commence this knotty task in the next chapters by briefly reviewing the history of child protection practice and we then consider some of the ways that jurisdictions have faced the many issues that confront them as they manage the enormity of the seemingly impossible challenge of protecting children, guaranteeing their safety, and ensuring they achieve their maximum potential.

Part II

The successes and failures of child protection

2 The chequered history of contemporary child protection practice

The period since the (re)discovery of child abuse in the early 1960s has been one where child protection policy and practice in all countries in the Anglophone world has been subject to conflicting demands and increasingly high profile political and media opprobrium. Child protection systems have been subject to continual change and reform, often in the wake of a major child abuse scandal, usually where a child has died and where a variety of health, welfare, and criminal justice agencies are seen to have failed to intervene appropriately. Social workers, in particular, have come in for considerable criticism and have not been seen as competent in fulfilling the tasks expected of them. Policy and practice have been changed primarily in response to failure and in a context of crisis. This is powerfully illustrated in the political response to the tragic death of Victoria Climbié in London in 2000.

Victoria Adjo Climbié was born near Abidjan in the Ivory Coast on November 2, 1991 and was the fifth of seven children. In 1998 she travelled with her aunt, Marie Therese Kouao, to Paris where they stayed for approximately 5 months, arriving in London on April 24, 1999. On April 26 they visited a Homeless Person's Unit as they needed somewhere to live. In the following eleven months Victoria, then called Anna, was known to four different social services departments in London, three housing authorities, two police child protection teams, two hospitals, and an NSPCC (National Society for the Prevention of Cruelty to Children) family center. Yet, when she died, on February 25, 2000, the Home Office pathologist found the cause of death to be hypothermia, which had arisen in the context of malnourishment, a damp environment, and restricted movement. He also found 128 separate injuries on her body as a result of being beaten by a range of sharp and blunt instruments. No part of her body had been spared. Marks on her wrists and ankles indicated that her arms and legs had been tied together. It was the worst case of deliberate harm to a child he had ever seen. Marie Therese Kouao and her boyfriend Carl Manning were charged with her murder and convicted on January 12, 2001. Sentencing them to life imprisonment, Judge Richard Hawkins told the pair that Anna had "died at both your hands a lonely drawn-out death," and added "lessons must be learned about the failures of social services and police." It was only after the conviction that it became known that Anna's real name was Victoria.

Alan Milburn, the then Minister of Health, led a wave of anguished reaction and said "she was undoubtedly failed repeatedly by the child protection system" and immediately ordered an urgent statutory public inquiry to be chaired by Lord Laming. This was to be the latest of many such inquiries in the UK since the public inquiry into the death of Maria Colwell in 1973 (Secretary of State for Social Services 1974), and when presenting Lord Laming's report (Laming 2003) to the House of Commons on January 28, 2003, Alan Milburn said:

> It is an all too familiar cry. In the past few decades there have been dozens of inquiries into awful cases of abuse and neglect. Each has called on us to learn the lesson of what went wrong. Indeed there is a remarkable consistency in both what went wrong and what is advocated to put it right.
>
> (Hansard, January 28, col 739)

This theme, of the failure to learn the lessons of the many public inquiries of the previous 30 years, and the need for fundamental change, was a central one which was picked up in the ensuing political debate and the media coverage of the Laming Report. The comment in the *Daily Mail* on January 29, 2003 was typical:

> Thirty years ago Britain was shocked when seven-year-old Maria Colwell was beaten to death by the stepfather. Then too, there was utter determination that such tragedies would never happen again. Yet despite other victims and inquiries since, have the fundamentals really been learned? Hardly.

The government responded with a Green Paper entitled *Every Child Matters* (Chief Secretary to the Treasury 2003) and embarked on the most fundamental "transformation" of children's services in England for over a generation (Parton 2006a,b). While, as we will argue, these changes are probably the most radical of any introduced by any Anglophone government, this process of tragic death, public inquiry, sense of outrage, new policies, and (sometimes) new legislation has been replicated across North America, Australasia, and the United Kingdom over this 30-year period.

However, this sense of crisis has not only arisen because of high profile tragedies. Resources have also been overstretched so that child protection systems have been working beyond capacity such that there has been a failure to provide appropriate support to parents, families, and children who need it. Any child protection system operating in a liberal democracy has to walk a fine tightrope. Not only is it important that children are protected, but that the privacy of the family should not be undermined. These are not only important issues for children, parents, and professionals, but also for the state itself which, while it must be able to protect the vulnerable and weak, must not undermine the more general freedoms of parents to bring children up in the ways they see as most appropriate. It is important that the state is not experienced and seen as a nanny state or an authoritarian state.

How different jurisdictions have addressed these issues has taken a number of different routes since the early 1960s, and it is to these that we now turn. However, the sense of crisis in child protection in the full glare of the media has never been far away. What are the various elements of this sense of crisis? How has it come about? And how have the various jurisdictions tried to respond? These are the key questions which this chapter will begin to address. The questions will be explored further in Chapter 3.

The original discovery of child abuse and its subsequent disappearance

For a phenomenon to take on the guise of a social problem requiring some form of state intervention, it first has to be defined and constituted as such, and the late nineteenth and early twentieth centuries are in many respects the period which provided the foundations of what was to become "the child protection system." What Linda Gordon (1989) calls the era of "nineteenth century child-saving" (p. 20) lasted until World War I, at which point child abuse effectively disappeared as a subject of social concern, until it was "rediscovered" by American paediatricians as the "battered child syndrome" nearly half a century later.

The first organized group of "child-savers," the New York Society for the Prevention of Cruelty to Children (SPCC), was formed in 1874 in response to the well-publicized case of Mary Ellen, who was the victim of severe physical abuse by her stepmother. Taking its approach (and name) from the animal welfare movement founded in England 50 years earlier, the SPCC's focus was on "rescuing" children from cruel and abusive parents. The "child rescue" movement arose at a time when children were first coming to be seen as priceless and vulnerable individuals and when women were finding their voices as uniquely qualified advocates for children and families (Gordon 1994; Zelizer 1994; Parker 1995). Soon there were chapters in other US states, along with new local and state agencies to address the problem.

Similar organizations were also established in England and Australia. For example, the first Society for the Prevention of Cruelty to Children was established in England in 1883. The NSPCC was formed in 1889 and was hugely successful in organizing the public and political campaign which produced the first legislation in England specifically to outlaw child cruelty, and give public agencies powers to protect children within their home and remove them if necessary—the 1889 Prevention of Cruelty to Children Act (Behlmer 1982; Parton 1985). While the image and rhetoric was very much concerned with "child rescue," as Ferguson (2004) has demonstrated from his detailed analysis of NSPCC case files in the north east of England, this was not the first option. NSPCC inspectors worked ostentatiously in the homes of poor communities describing, classifying and assigning deviancy. Here were "social actors actively constructing the foundations of modern forms of knowledge, of therapeutic and cultural practice: in short, a professional culture that would take child protection into the twentieth century" (Ferguson 1990: 135). Indeed, many of the dilemmas of modern practice were present as inspectors advocated for clients, pondered the advisability of rehabilitating children, and sought to reform and change parents (Ferguson 2004). From the outset, the newly established child protection services faced a significant challenge which was a central dilemma in any liberal society, namely: how can a legal basis be devised for the power to intervene into the privacy of the family in order to protect children in a way which does not undermine the institution of the family and convert all families into clients of the state? (Parton 1991). Three inter-related issues have therefore always provided the context for child protection services: the primacy of parents vis-à-vis the child protection system; the scope of government intervention; and the nature of government intervention (Waldfogel 1998: 71). The balance in the way these three issues are addressed, however, will vary according to the changing demands and political, economic and social/cultural contexts in which they are located.

However, after 1918, much of this high profile activity and focus virtually disappeared from public view and became primarily an issue to be addressed locally and on a case-by-case basis. A number of explanations have been suggested for this. For example, in relation to England, Parker (1995) has argued that the decline in the women's movement following the granting of universal suffrage and changes in the NSPCC, to whom the government was happy to leave the day-to-day responsibility for child cruelty, became more bureaucratic and less campaigning, and was less willing to publicize the deaths of children at the hands of their parents (Ferguson 1996, 1997).

In the US, the federal government established the Children's Bureau in 1912 but child abuse was not high on its agenda. While the Bureau was the primary federal agency for strengthening family life (Halpern 1991), its primary focus was upon improving and rationalizing financial and other forms of assistance for children and families. To this end, the outcome of the Social Security Act 1935 was to lodge "public assistance" programs for families with the Social Security Board and "child welfare services" with the Children's Bureau (Hanlon 1966).

In England, the Children Act 1948, which created local authority Children's Departments and abolished the last remains of the hated Poor Law, was prompted in part by an inquiry into the much publicized death of a foster child in 1945 (Monckton 1945). However, the focus was not upon child abuse in the family, for the priority was on improving the circumstances of children "deprived of a normal home life" and who were living in, often institutionalized, residential care. More generally, the changes aimed to usher in a new, more enlightened age which aimed to prevent children coming into care and helping families stay together after the terrible experiences of war and evacuation.

Children's Departments attempted to establish, for the first time in England, a professional state-sponsored *child welfare* service which saw the family as an object of positive social policy (Packman 1981). The aim was not to punish bad parents but to act in the interests of children. As the emphasis was on the strength and formative power of the natural, nuclear family this meant trying to maintain children in their family (Holman 1996). It heralded an era where families, primarily mothers, who came to the attention of children's departments, were encouraged and helped to care for their own children in their own homes, which underlined the importance of both the home and the child's parents (again primarily mothers) to his or her development. The practice of local authority social work with children and families during the post-war period, up until the early 1970s, was thus imbued with a considerable optimism, for it was believed that measured and significant improvements could be made in the lives of individuals and families via judicious, professional interventions. Child welfare social work operated quietly and confidently and in a relatively uncontested way, which reflected a supportive social mandate. It was allowed wide professional discretion and the family was assumed to be an essentially beneficent, "natural" and consensual institution where the interests of parents (both mothers and fathers) were in harmony and had the interests and welfare of their children at heart. Such a conception was essentially based on a predominantly white, middle-class (or respectable working-class) model of the nuclear family where children were born in wedlock and lived with their parents throughout childhood.

The high point of this optimistic growth of social work in its approach to child welfare in England, came with the establishment of the larger and more wide-ranging social services departments which superseded children's departments in 1971, and which aimed to provide a *family* service. It reflected the belief that social problems could be overcome, via state intervention, by professional experts drawing on social scientific knowledge and using their skills in relationships, and envisaged a progressive, universal service available to all and with wide community support.

While similar assumptions were at play in other Anglophone societies at the time, it is notable that significant sections of the population did not share these characteristics. Parents were much more likely to be in potential conflict with child welfare agencies and their children considerably over-represented in the population who were taken into care. This was most evident in relation to children of color in the UK and North America (Shireman 2003) and, in particular, Indigenous children in Australia, New Zealand, and North America (Johnston 1983; Cunneen and Libesman 2000; Shireman 2003; Love 2006). Indeed, the longstanding policies and practices for Indigenous families and children have had such profound effects on these communities that they have been identified as tantamount to cultural genocide by some (Churchill 1994; Neu and Therrien 2003).

Historically, the grossly disproportionate numbers of Indigenous children in child welfare systems, including Australian Aborigines and Torres Strait

Islanders, New Zealand Maoris, Canadian First Nations people, Métis and Inuit, and US Native Americans, is only partly explained by their significant economic, social and health disadvantage. Across these nations, institutionalized racism and colonization have also led to a range of destructive practices such as assimilation, child removal and widespread adoption into white families, and oppression via schooling regimes that entailed enforced residentials, tried to remove native language and transmission of cultural practices, and had profound effects on people's collective and individual identities. For many, the end result has been mental health problems, and alcohol and substance abuse, and suicide. In a poignant piece, Johnston describes the irony present in suicide of First Nations people who have previously been in care "Christian believes that his brother's death was the result of his treatment by the child welfare system. Actions ostensibly taken 'in the best interests of the child' may have shortened his life" (Johnston 1983: xx).

There have been a host of inquiries into these practices and the current plight of Indigenous people, for example, the *Bringing them Home Report*, which documented the terrible experiences of the "Stolen Generation" in Australia, and the ongoing trauma experienced by those directly involved and subsequent generations (Human Rights and Equal Opportunity Commission (HREOC) 1997). A range of indicators establish that, compared to other members of the society, Indigenous people generally experience significant disadvantage, including poor housing and high unemployment, poverty, lower educational achievements, increased family violence, higher likelihood of being in prison or in contact with the criminal justice system, and susceptibility to a range of debilitating illnesses, resulting in them dying a lot younger (Cunneen and Libesman 2000; Shireman 2003; Freymond and Cameron 2006; Cheers *et al.* 2007). Moreover, these contemporary difficulties continue to bring Indigenous children and families to the attention of child protection authorities disproportionately.

Child welfare systems have attempted to alter this state of affairs, including via legislation that emphasizes preservation of cultural and familial ties such as the US 1978 Child Welfare Act (Shireman 2003). Nevertheless, the difficulties in changing mainstream child protection organizational and individual worker's practices to make them culturally congruent and appropriate are significant (Ross 1992). There have been a number of progressive attempts to redress these circumstances made by a range of Indigenous communities in all countries, including self-determination policies, reparations for past wrongs (e.g. Canada's Common Experience Payment), funding and resources for Indigenous-run organizations, and developing innovative programs and other measures to help communities regain control over their lives (Freymond and Cameron 2006). Many Indigenous people have trained in social work and other disciplines, making a significant difference (Hill 2000; Zapf *et al.* 2003). Although there have been some important successes, the fact remains that while child protection systems attempt to strengthen Indigenous family and community systems, the net effect is often the opposite (Johnston 1983).

The (re)emergence of child abuse as a major social problem

Throughout the 1940s and 1950s articles in US medical journals were identifying trauma to children which appeared to be intentionally inflicted by caregivers (Igraham and Matson 1944; Smith 1944; Caffey 1946; Silverman 1953; Wooley and Evans 1955; Bakwin 1956; Jones and Davis 1957; Friedman 1958; Miller 1959). However, it was Kempe *et al.*'s identification of the "battered child syndrome" in 1962 which catapulted the issue of child abuse back onto professional, public and political agendas in the US (Kempe *et al.* 1962). The idea was quickly "imported" into the UK via the NSPCC and a number of medical and social work professionals (see Parton 1985 for a detailed analysis of the process) and also Australia (Scott and Swain 2002). As a consequence, policy and practice in the entire Anglophone world was tremendously influenced by the original conceptualization of the problem in the US and what were seen as the best ways of responding.

Unlike the original nineteenth century "discovery," it was medical professionals, rather than victims, survivors, community groups and the women's movement who not only brought the issue back to public attention but, in the process, conceptualized it in very particular ways. It was defined as a "syndrome" or "disease" and, hence, was professionalized, doctors being seen as the experts in "diagnosis." It is quite clear that the term "battered child syndrome" was specifically chosen by Kempe *et al.*, as opposed to "physical abuse," in order to appeal to as wide an audience as possible, particularly conservative paediatricians. Kempe *et al.* wanted no hint of legal, social or deviancy dimensions—the problem was *medicalized* and medical experts and medical technology, such as the X-ray, were seen as key in identifying what would otherwise be hidden injuries.

The article identified what seemed to be a quite specific and particular condition which was found in young children, usually under three, who had experienced *serious physical abuse*. The paper argued that the syndrome was a significant cause of childhood disability and death, and that the syndrome was often misdiagnosed but should be considered in any child showing evidence of possible trauma or neglect, or where there was a marked discrepancy between the clinical findings and the story presented by parents. The use of X-rays to aid "diagnosis" was stressed, and it was argued that the prime concern of the physician was to make the correct "diagnosis", and to make certain that a similar event did not occur again. The authors recommended that doctors should report all incidents to law enforcement or child protection agencies. It was also said that the problem was not simply concerned with poverty, and that the characteristics of the parents were that: "they are immature, impulsive, self-centered, hypersensitive and quick to react with poorly controlled aggression" (Kempe *et al.* 1962: 19). Both the article and the approach were to have an enormous influence on the way child abuse was thought about and responded to for many years to come.

There was an immediate impact in the US. In 1963 the Children's Bureau issued a model reporting law whereby certain health and welfare professionals would be required to report cases of actual and suspected child abuse to designated public authorities, and all fifty US states had adopted such laws by 1967 (Hutchison 1993). This was followed by the first national child protection legislation, the Child Abuse and Prevention and Treatment Act (CAPTA) in 1974, which, among other things, required states to have such laws in place. Nelson (1984) has suggested three primary reasons as to why the issue was responded to so quickly. First, child abuse was seen as a clear value issue; that children should not be abused or neglected was not seen as controversial and no one wanted to be seen as opposing such a development. Second, the issue was narrowly framed; for although the CAPTA definition included both abuse and neglect, the primary focus in the public and legislative debates was on battered children as opposed, for example, to children living in less than optimal situations. Third, the issue appeared to have a simple and inexpensive solution; requiring doctors and other named professionals who had frequent contact with children to report instances of abuse to the named public authorities. Essentially, it was assumed that child abuse and neglect, conceptualized in terms of "the battered child syndrome," was a specific and small-scale problem but which had horrendous consequences for some, particularly very young children, and that this could be addressed by the introduction of a new, statutorily based, system of reporting. It would have minor financial and professional consequences.

Just over 10 years later, a similar process took place in Australia. In 1977, New South Wales was the first Australian state to pass comparable legislation and other states followed, so that all Australian states now have some form of mandatory child abuse reporting laws (Ainsworth 2002), with Western Australia only recently legislating for requisite reporting of child sexual abuse by authorities following the recommendations of the Ford Report (Ford 2007).

While the introduction of mandatory reporting legislation has been particularly associated with the growing problems with child protection systems in the Anglophone world, it is also clear that the problems are not resolvable simply by abolishing mandatory reporting. The problems are much more fundamental. As we will demonstrate later, the UK has never had a mandatory reporting system, yet has had similar challenges to those experienced in the US and Australia. The problems have emanated, first, because of the assumptions underpinning child protection systems from the outset, and, second, because of a number of social changes which have had a particular impact upon anxieties about children and the institution of childhood more generally.

As Gary Melton (2005) has argued, the original designers of modern child protection systems made two interconnected and fundamental errors, and both could be seen to emanate from assumptions which underpinned the notion of "the battered child syndrome." Both the *scope* and the *complexity* of the problem of child abuse and neglect were underestimated.

The assumption early in the history of the modern child protection system was that the problem of child maltreatment was reducible to "syndromes" —in effect, that abusive and neglecting parents were either very sick or very evil and that they could thus be appropriately characterized as "those people" who were fundamentally different from ourselves . . . Although such cases do occur, they are relatively rare. Most cases involve neglect . . . further, searches for distinctive behavioral syndromes have proven elusive.

(Melton 2005: 11)

The original failure to recognize both the scope and complexity of the problem was exacerbated by the subsequent considerable broadening of the concept of child abuse, or child maltreatment as it was increasingly referred to in the US. While the notion of the "battered child syndrome" proved the dominant underlying metaphor for many years, the category of child abuse was also subject to various "mouldings" (Hacking 1988, 1991, 1992) and "diagnostic inflation" (Dingwall 1989: 29) so that by the late 1980s it included emotional abuse, neglect, and sexual abuse, as well as physical abuse and was no longer focused only on young children but included young people up to the age of 18.

At the same time, the social context in which this broadening in the category of child abuse was taking place was itself in a state of considerable flux. Dorothy Scott (2006a) has identified two "drivers" which she sees as important in influencing policy and practice: the idea of the child as a holder of human rights, and the notion of the child as a psychological being. She argues that the view of the child as a holder of human rights has grown over the past 30 years and that this has placed increased expectations on the state to uphold the rights of the child. While this may be a factor in some jurisdictions, it is likely to have been less influential in the US, which is one of just two countries that have not signed the Convention of the Rights of the Child. Second, she sees the broadening definition as very much reflecting the growing recognition that harm to children is also caused by psychological and emotional factors as much as, if not more so, by physical acts.

In addition, however, and as one of us has argued extensively elsewhere (Parton 2006a), the last thirty years have also witnessed other considerable social changes. The changing nature of "the family" and communities, particularly under the impact of growing globalization, has led to an increased sense of risk and social anxiety, which are seen to have major implications and consequences for children. It is not only children themselves but the institution of childhood itself which is seen as being under threat.

The loss of traditional families embedded within secure communities and the growth in the individualization of social life (Beck and Beck-Gernsheim 2002) creates a context in which there is a greater emotional investment in children in what seems a more uncertain and less safe world. Thus, what increasingly happens to children seems to symbolize the key benchmarks for the kind of society we have become, and a primary focus for the aspirations, projections and longings on the part of adults. Children can thus be seen to envision a "nostalgia" or longing for more secure times now past (Jenks 1996), together with a growing investment in the future in order to bring about a better world. Adults have become so concerned about the safety of children because "children have become our principal concern, we have become their protectors and nurturers and they have become our primary love objects, our human capital and our future" (Jenks 1996: 99). Whatever the specific or more general reasons, there is no doubt that by the late 1980s the number of reports to child protection agencies had increased exponentially and the sense of crisis in child protection systems had become pervasive.

The growing crisis in child protection

The dramatic increase in official reports suggested that the number of children suffering or at risk of child abuse was much larger than assumed when the new child protection systems were set up. At the same time, while the numbers were increasing, a decreasing proportion was deemed to be "substantiated."

In the US the number of official reports of child abuse increased from 9,563 in 1967 to 669,000 in 1976, to over 2 million in 1987, and over 3 million in 1994 (Figure 2.1). However, while the proportion of cases "substantiated" or "indicated" was over 60 percent in the 1970s, this figure had dropped to under 40 percent by the late 1980s. The exact meaning of the terms "substantiated"

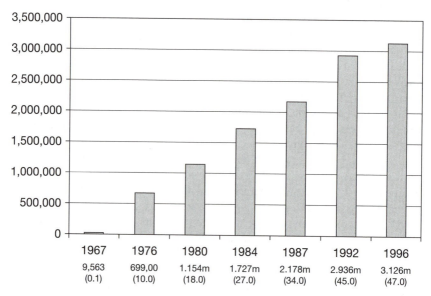

Figure 2.1 Child abuse and neglect reports in the United States (selected years, 1967–1996). Rate per 100,000 in brackets.

Source: Waldfogel 1998; Parton *et al.* 1997.

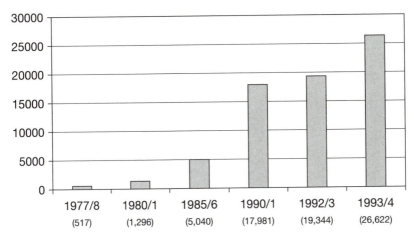

Figure 2.2 Notifications of child abuse and neglect, Department of Health and Community Services, Victoria.

Source: Parton *et al.* 1997.

and "indicated" varies somewhat between states, but generally a "substantiated" case is one in which the investigating social worker has found a reasonable cause to believe that a child has been abused or neglected, or is at elevated risk of abuse or neglect, while an "indicated" case is one in which there is some evidence that abuse or neglect has occurred but in which the evidence does not meet the threshold for "substantiation" (Waldfogel 1998).

Similar trends were evident in Canada (Trocme *et al.* 1995; Swift 1997) but were, perhaps, even more marked in Australia. While the way statistics are collated varies between states, similar patterns were very evident; but, partly because Australian states introduced their child protection systems about 10 years later than the US, the rate of growth in reports/notifications was even more evident. For example, in the state of Victoria notifications of child abuse and neglect increased more than 5,000 percent between 1977/8 and 1993/4 (Figure 2.2). Indeed, since the middle 1990s, and into the new millennium, this trend has continued with further staggering increases of notifications in Australia (Ainsworth and Hansen 2006; D. Scott 2006a; E. Scott 2006).

In England there are no comparable statistics. While it is estimated that in 1992 there were about 160,000 child protection reports (requiring a Section 47 investigation) (Department of Health 1995), there has not been a systematic attempt to collect and collate statistics on child protection reports/notifications as there has been in the US and Australia. The only statistics available which cover the last quarter of the twentieth century relate to child protection registers. A child's name is placed on the register where, following an investigation and a multidisciplinary case conference, it is felt that the child has been and/or continues to be at risk of suffering abuse or neglect and is subject to a "child protection plan."

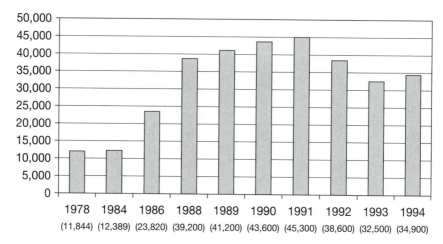

Figure 2.3 Numbers of children on child protection registers in England (selected years, 1978–1994).

Source: Parton *et al.* 1997: 5.

Figure 2.3 indicates that the numbers of children on child protection registers in England quadrupled between 1978 and 1991, but declined by a quarter between 1991 and 1993 following the Department of Health's strong recommendation that the category of "grave concern" should be dropped from the register.

By the early 1990s a number of authoritative reports were arguing that child protection systems were, at best, out of balance or, at worst, in crisis and were in need of considerable rationalization and/or reform. For example, the US Advisory Board on Child Abuse and Neglect (US ABCAN) (1990) commented that:

> The most serious shortcomings of the nation's system of intervention on behalf of children is that it depends on reporting and response processes that has punitive connotations and requires massive resources dedicated to the investigation of allegations. State and County child welfare programs have not been designed to get immediate help to families based on voluntary requests for assistance. As a result, it has become far easier to pick up the telephone to report one's neighbor for child abuse than it is for that neighbor to pick up the telephone and receive help before the abuse happens.
>
> (US ABCAN 1990: 80)

And 3 years later:

> The result of the current design of the child protection system is that investigation often seems to occur for its own sake, without any realistic

hope of meaningful treatment to prevent the recurrence of maltreatment or to ameliorate its effects, even if the report of suspected maltreatment is validated.

(US ABCAN 1993: 10–11)

It seems that the child protection systems had developed wide "nets" in which were caught a whole variety of concerns about children, and that certain sections of the population were at greater risk of being caught in the nets than others. Waldfogel (1998) demonstrated that over half of all reports in the US were neglect cases and that, although the children reported to child protection agencies were a diverse group, those from racial and ethnic minorities were disproportionately represented, as were children from lone-mother families and poor families. In 1996, over 40 percent of children reported to child protection agencies were from racial or ethnic minority groups: 27 percent were African American, 11 percent were Latino, 2 percent were Native American, 1 percent was Asian, and 2 percent were from other minority groups. However, it seemed that low income and poverty, rather than race and ethnicity, were the prime determinants of the higher rates at which minority children were reported to child protection agencies (Waldfogel 1998). While the reasons for this were likely to be diverse, they included the fact that poorer families, parents, and children came into greater contact with a range of health, welfare and criminal justice agencies and were also living in high stress contexts which required greater help and support, and a major route to access to resources was via the child protection system. An investigatory response, however, may not be appropriate for all these situations, particularly where the nature of the concerns related to child neglect. What was also becoming clear in the US was that a considerable amount of energy was being expended in not just deciding whether a case was "substantiated" or not, but in deciding which cases could be allocated a service and, more generally, investing time and resources in managing the child protection system itself. The allocation of scarce "child welfare" resources was being dominated by a narrowly focused, forensically driven and crisis-orientated "child protection" system (Kamerman and Khan 1990).

Similar findings were emerging in other jurisdictions. The research carried out by David Thorpe in Western Australia (Thorpe 1994) is particularly instructive in this respect and, as we will demonstrate in Chapter 3, was to prove influential in informing policy and practice changes in Western Australia in the 1990s. Thorpe collected data on a 100 percent sample of reports (655 reports) to three of Western Australia's Department for Community Services area offices, where there were allegations of child abuse and neglect between January 1 and March 31, 1987 and the case files analyzed for the subsequent 52 weeks. After investigation, just 33 percent (216) of the reports were considered to concern abused children, while a further 16.6 percent (109) were judged to be "at risk" of abuse or neglect (see Figure 2.4). Despite these assessments, just 27 percent (178) cases received a service, of which 9.7 percent

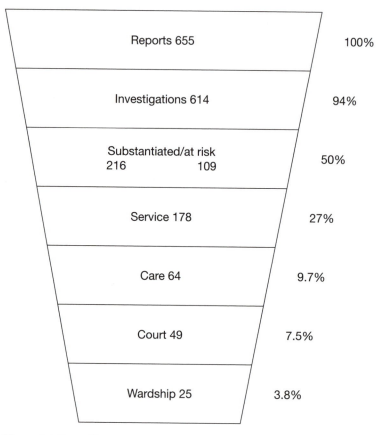

Figure 2.4 Funnelling and filtering child abuse reports in Western Australia.
Source: Parton *et al.* 1997.

(64) were taken into care. The proportion of the original 655 reports taken to the Children's Court on "care and protection" grounds was less than 10 percent, while just 3.8 percent (25 children) were made state wards. Of the allegations, 42.1 percent related to single female parent households and 7 percent to single male parents, while 23 percent related to Aboriginal children. This "over-representation" of both single parent and Aboriginal households was evident in the careers of the children throughout the child protection process during the 52-week period analyzed, and was even more evident in a more detailed analysis carried out by Thorpe a few years later (Thorpe 1997).

Thorpe carried out a much smaller replication of the study, again based on a 100 percent sample (100 files) in a local authority in South Wales three years later, and found a very similar pattern both in the make up of the families (48 percent single parents) and also in the way the child protection system operated in filtering out cases (Figure 2.5).

While a similar "crisis" was developing in England, the process whereby this emerged and the context in which it happened was somewhat different. Up until 1987 there had been numerous high profile tragedies of children dying at the hands of their parents or carers while under the supervision of social workers, since the death of Maria Colwell in 1973 (Secretary of State 1974). Between the publication of the Maria Colwell inquiry report and 1985, there were twenty-nine further inquiries into the deaths of children as a result of abuse (Corby *et al.* 1998). There was a remarkable similarity in the findings (DHSS 1982). Most identified:

•   a lack of interdisciplinary communication;
•   a lack of properly trained and experienced front-line workers;
•   inadequate supervision; and
•   too little focus on the needs of the children as distinct from those of the parents.

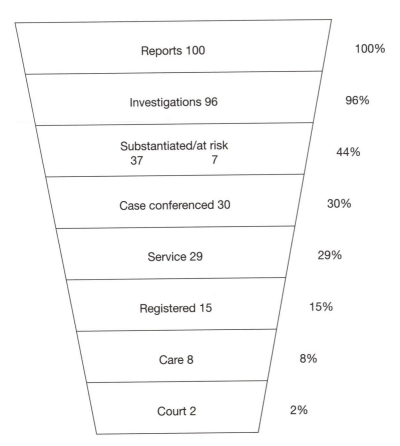

Figure 2.5 Funnelling and filtering child abuse reports in a South Wales authority.
Source: Parton *et al.* 1997.

The overriding concern was a lack of coordination between the various agencies and a failure to identify and respond to abuse. Throughout the period, central government responded by producing ever more detailed procedures and guidance as to how to handle child abuse cases.

However, the intense public and media interest reached a new peak in the mid 1980s with three high profile inquiries into the deaths of children in three London boroughs (London Borough of Brent 1985; London Borough of Lambeth 1987; London Borough of Greenwich 1987). All the children had died as a result of physical abuse and had suffered neglect, and the child care professionals, particularly social workers, were perceived as having failed to protect the children. The professionals were seen as too naïve and sentimental with parents, failed to concentrate on the interests of the children, and to use the statutory authority vested in them. As a consequence, they did too little, too late. The emphasis in the inquiry reports' recommendations was to encourage social workers to use their legal mandate to intervene in families to protect children, rationalize the multidisciplinary framework to enhance coordination, and improve practitioners' knowledge of the signs and symptoms of child abuse so that it could be spotted in day-to-day practice (see Parton 1991, Chapter 3). Such recommendations very much reflected the thrust of policy and practice change of the previous 15 years. However, while central government was in the process of revising its guidance to take account of these most recent public inquiries, an exceptional child abuse scandal exploded into the media and introduced a public and political debate of a very different order.

The Cleveland "affair" broke in the summer of 1987 and was focused on the activities of two paediatricians and social workers in a hospital in Middlesbrough, a declining chemical and industrial town in the north-east of England. During a period of a few weeks, over a hundred children were removed from their families to an emergency place of safety (the hospital) on the basis of what was seen by the media (Franklin 1989), and two local Members of Parliament (Bell 1988), as questionable diagnoses of child sexual abuse. A public inquiry was established by the Secretary of State for Social Services, and reported the following year (Secretary of State 1988).

Not only was this the first scandal and public inquiry into possible overreaction by professionals, it was also the first on sexual abuse, and the first when medical science, as well as social work, was put under close scrutiny (Parton 1991; Ashenden 1996, 2004). Unlike most developments up until this point, which had very much carried the imprint of thinking in the US, developments in Cleveland were a very British affair and had a history and impact, both in Britain and abroad, of their own (Hacking 1991, 1992).

It is in this context that we need to understand the Children Act 1989. While the Act was not a simple reaction to child abuse inquiries, it was very much concerned with trying to construct a better balance, not just between the rights and responsibilities of individuals and agencies, but between the need to protect children and the need to enable parents to challenge intervention in the upbringing of their children (Parton 1991, Chapter 6). It was, perhaps, the first attempt in the Anglophone world to carry out a serious critical appraisal of the impact of the child protection system(s) which had been developed since the mid 1960s.

The central principles of the Act encouraged an approach to child welfare based on *negotiation* with families, and involving parents and children in agreed plans. The accompanying guidance and regulations encouraged professionals to work in *partnership* with parents and young people. Similarly, the Act, particularly under Section 17, encouraged a role for the state which would *support* "children in need" at an early stage, thus reducing the need for care proceedings and emergency interventions. In the process, it attempted to keep to a minimum the situations where social workers would rely upon a policing and investigatory approach dominated by a focus upon a narrowly defined forensic concern, and put in its place an emphasis on providing help and support with the full agreement of parents and children.

This attempt to "refocus" children's services was reinforced a few years later by the publication of the Audit Commission report (1994) *Seen But Not Heard: Coordinating Community Health and Social Services for Children in Need* and the launch by the Department of Health of *Child Protection: Messages from Research* (Department of Health 1995). The latter was to prove of particular importance in both reinforcing these themes and trying to take policy and practice in a new direction. The report summarized over twenty research studies into the processes and outcomes of child protection interventions in England in the early 1990s; thirteen of the studies had been funded by the Department of Health following the fallout from the Cleveland inquiry and the apparent confusion in the reactions of the investigating agencies (Parton 1997). The report argued that while there was little evidence that children were being missed and suffering unnecessarily, as implied by most child abuse public inquiries, and therefore was "successful," according to a narrow definition of child protection, this was at a cost. Many of the children and parents involved felt alienated and angry. There was an overemphasis on forensic concerns and there was far too much time and resources spent on investigations and not enough on developing longer term coordinated treatment and preventive strategies. More specifically, it called for a "rebalancing" or "refocusing" in child protection which would prioritize Section 17 and Part 3 of the Children Act 1989, in terms of supporting families with "children in need," and thereby keep notions of policing and coercive intervention to a minimum. It similarly suggested that Section 47 of the Act should be understood as a duty to *inquire*, rather than simply a forensically determined power to investigate.

Both the Audit Commission report and *Messages from Research* (Department of Health 1995) were considerably influenced by the study carried out by Gibbons *et al.* (1995). This research, based in eight local authorities and carried out over a 16-week period in 1992, identified all children referred for a new child protection investigation (1,888 cases) and tracked their progress through the child protection system for up to 26 weeks via social work records and case conference minutes. What was seen as particularly significant was the way a series of *filters* and *funnels* operated (see Figure 2.6). At the first level, 26 percent of referrals were filtered out by social work staff at the duty stage after initial checks without any direct contact with the child or family. At the second, the investigation itself, another 50 percent were filtered out and never reached an initial case conference. Of the remainder, just 15 percent were placed on a child protection register. Thus, six out of every seven children who entered the child protection system were filtered out without their names being placed on the register.

Of allegations, 49 percent were "not substantiated", and the investigation led to no further action in a high proportion (44 percent of those investigated). There were no interventions to protect the child nor were any services provided. In only 4 percent of all cases referred were children removed from home on a statutory order at any time during the study. The study also found that over one-third (36 percent) of the total referrals were headed by a lone parent, and in only 30 percent of cases were both natural parents living in the

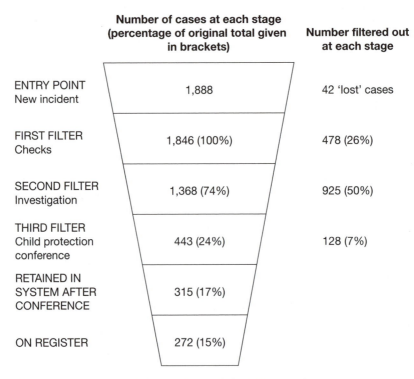

Figure 2.6 Operation of filters in the English child protection system.
Source: Gibbons *et al.* 1995.

same household, while 57 percent lacked a wage earner and 54 percent were dependent on income support. It was the most vulnerable sections of the population who were most likely to become the object of the child protection system.

The findings in relation to neglect were particularly illuminating. Of the 392 (100 percent) referrals for suspected neglect, 40 percent were filtered out at the first stage, 46 percent filtered out at the second stage after investigation, so that just 14 percent reached a case conference, with just 6 percent being placed on the register. In 65 percent of all the neglect cases, the researchers could not identify any protective actions taken or any mobilization of support. Yet the researchers felt that the children had the highest number of poverty indicators and "just as many indicators of vulnerability as those referred for physical or sexual abuse. Thus the commonest picture was of children not reaching the threshold for child protection proceedings, but not getting any preventive help either" (Parton 1995: 85). The research by Gibbons *et al.* (1995) was the first time that any sort of map of the child protection system and how it operated had been available in England. While different in detail, it had many similarities to that in the US and Australia.

Conclusions

By the early/mid 1990s evidence was thus emerging in the US, Australia, and England that there were significant problems with their child protection systems. Public inquiries, authoritative official reports and research—while different in detail and emphasis—were all pointing to significant problems which needed to be addressed. Some commentators argued that the problems arose because the definitions of child abuse and neglect were too vague and all inclusive, leading to an "over-reporting" of cases such that the system was unable to cope. What was required was a narrowing of state intervention and a much tighter set of definitions as to what sort of cases should be reported (Besharov 1988, 1990). Others argued that the much bigger problem was not "over-reporting" but that agencies did not seem to have sufficient resources, and therefore failed to provide children with a sensitive and effective response (Finkelhor 1990).

In the light of the growing consensus in the US that the child protection system was in need of a major overhaul, the Harvard Executive Session on Child Protective Services was convened in 1994 to consider ways forward. It was felt that there were five major problems with the US child protection system—and all of the problems could be seen to apply to other Anglophone systems at that time (Waldfogel 1998; 2008).

The first problem was *over-inclusion*, whereby some children and families were included, while others who were low risk were subject to an unnecessarily adversarial and forensic investigation. At the same time, and second, there was *under-inclusion*, whereby some children and families that should be involved within the child protection system were not. This may have been because they were missed and not reported, or because families asked for voluntary assistance at an early stage of difficulty but did not meet the threshold for inclusion. The third problem, which both reflected and arose from the first two was *capacity*. The number of reports had increased so dramatically over the previous 30 years that the number of children and families involved far exceeded the capacity of the system to serve them.

The fourth problem was, what Waldfogel called, *service delivery*, for even if children and families did manage to cross the threshold for inclusion appropriately, many did not receive the right sort of service or, in many cases, any service at all. The fifth problem is to do with *service orientation*. In being so concerned to investigate cases of child abuse there was a failure to engage with children and families and try to address their particular needs. In addition, such an orientation was not only stigmatizing and antagonistic to those it confronted, it also acted to discourage others—both families and professionals —from making referrals where there may be a need for help and support. Typically, child protection systems provided a narrowly prescribed response to reports of abuse and neglect, so that reports that were screened must be investigated according to certain clearly defined rules and procedures and according to strict time frames.

Waldfogel and her colleagues argued that the only way to overcome these problems was by a "paradigm shift" and in terms of the development of a "differential response" model. Such a model had a number of similarities to those being developed in England and parts of Australia, and it is to these that we turn in the next chapter. As we will see, a number of the principles which informed the English Children Act 1989, and the attempts to reform policy and practice following the "refocusing debate," are evident in these emerging new approaches.

3   Differential responses and
changing social mandates

From the early 1990s there was increasing debate about, and reform of, child protection systems in response to the growing criticisms and, in some jurisdictions, sense of crisis. Much of this was concerned with the development of a "differential response" approach which tried to move away from the narrow, forensically driven, investigatory approaches of the 1970s and 1980s. In many respects these new systems could be seen to reflect the concerns addressed in *Messages from Research*, which we discussed in the previous chapter. By the start of the new millennium, however, it was clear that, prompted by a whole range of concerns related to children, childhood, parenting, and "family" life more generally, a number of policy and practice initiatives wanted to go beyond the "differential response" approach. There were increasing efforts to develop broader, more holistic and integrated approaches where the current and future welfare and "well-being" of the child, not simply protecting them from harm, was the central focus. Such developments were not simply concerned with trying to integrate child protection and family approaches (Parton 1997), but had the overall health and development of the child as the focus. In the process, the balance between the rights and responsibilities of children, parents, professionals, and the state would be subject to significant reconfiguration. While such developments were evident in a number of jurisdictions, it is England which has embarked on the most radical transformation.

In many respects, however, the complexities and tensions in the work increase as a result. In broadening the focus and integrating a whole variety of systems and agencies, the demands upon front-line staff intensify. In particular, the introduction of various information and communication technologies, the demands for accountability, and the managerialization of the work have an enormous impact on the nature of the work (Parton 2007). While the language is increasingly framed in terms of improving children's "well-being," the context in which this takes place is dominated by ideas of performance management and an outcomes-driven business culture.

Differential response

In responding to the problems within existing child protection systems, "differential response" approaches aim to build a more comprehensive strategy for improving child protection. They aim to rethink and reframe the aims and assumptions of child protection. There has never been any doubt, however, that their focus is the reform of child protection. "Differential response" is a form of practice in child protection services that allows for more than one method of response to reports of child abuse and neglect. Also called "dual track," "multiple track," or "alternative response," the approach recognizes the variation in the nature of reports and the importance of responding differentially.

Waldfogel (1998) suggests three elements are key to the approach. First, it recognizes the diversity of families, and aims to provide case-specific assessments and service plans, in order to deliver a "customized response." Second, it does not envision one agency acting alone but calls for a community-based system where child protection services continue to play the lead role but work with other state, voluntary and private agencies to provide both preventive and protective services. Third, and perhaps most significantly for policy and practice development, it recognizes the importance of "family support" services in preventing child abuse and offering such services at a much earlier stage before the problems reach crisis proportions and before the child is abused or becomes at serious risk of abuse.

What became increasingly evident in the 1990s, particularly in the light of a number of international research projects which compared child protection policies and practices, was that there was wide variation in how this was carried out in different Western societies. More particularly, it seemed that systems which had followed the North American model were very different from those developed in Northern Europe and Scandinavia (see, for example, Cooper *et al.* 1995; Hetherington *et al.* 1997; Gilbert 1997; Harder and Pringle 1997; Pringle 1998; Hill *et al.* 2002; Khoo *et al.* 2002). As discussed in the previous chapter, for those which followed the North American model, the focus was the act or threatened act of abuse, and the primary intervention was in the form of a forensic investigation, which is often adversarial. In contrast, the more "family support" approach sees the problems as primarily arising from family conflict or dysfunction, which were seen to arise from social and psychological difficulties, which are usually responsive to public aid. Depending on the nature of the problems, cases were referred to a variety of agencies that provided support, counselling, advice, and therapy. The approach was essentially benign and aimed to be helpful. This is the dominant perspective in Northern Europe and Scandinavia.

"Differential response" draws on both approaches. It moves away from an incident-based, adversarial investigation for *all* reports, toward a more family and assessment approach for *some* reports, and aims to offer services to some families without having to investigate and substantiate the allegations. As originally envisaged, "differential response" focused on responding differentially to accepted reports of abuse, rather than those that had been screened out as inappropriate for child protection services. While "differential response" systems usually retain the potential for investigation as previously, the opportunity for offering a more holistic family assessment is also available and the preferred response wherever possible. Such an approach is based on a voluntary agreement and tends to be strength-based and community-oriented. It aims to minimize confrontation, enhance cooperation, and strengthen the family's ability to take care of itself. The focus is the assessment of need rather than the investigation of an incident. A number of US states have adopted the approach with a number of positive effects (English *et al.* 2000; US Department of Health and Human Services 2001, 2003; Daro *et al.* 2005; Johnson *et al.* 2005; Loman and Siegel 2005; Sawyer and Lohrbach 2005; Shusterman *et al.* 2005).

An early attempt to introduce a differential response system to child abuse reports occurred in Western Australia in 1996. Called *New Directions in Child Protection and Family Support*, it was developed following the research by David Thorpe in the late 1980s carried out in Western Australia, which we discussed in the previous chapter. In the context of increasing reports, reduced substantiation rates, decreasing departmental morale, and a general incapacity of the Department of Family and Children's Services to respond adequately to the increased child protection demands being made on it, *New Directions* was the name given to its new way of managing and responding to child abuse reports. There were a number of principles which informed the approach (Department of Family and Children's Services 1996):

- Recognition of the *importance of duty and intake processes* in terms of both the need for experienced and well-qualified staff to undertake the tasks and the importance of gathering quality information, which would assist in making accurate classifications and, hence, how the Department would respond.
- An emphasis on *professional judgment, assessment and supervision* rather than prescriptive procedures.
- Rather than the referrer (as previously), it would be departmental officers who would determine whether or not a report was a *child maltreatment allegation* (CMA), and in all such cases the senior designated officer must endorse the decision to classify the referral as a CMA.
- The introduction of a *new reason for contact classification* called a *child concern report* (CCR), which would be assigned to referrals where there was no indication of maltreatment, but concern was expressed about a child's welfare in relation to home environment, and where the precise nature of the problem was unclear and required further assessment. It was to function as a temporary classification, which was current only while an assessment was being conducted to determine the nature of the concern and what services, if any, were required. The introduction of the CCR was

a serious attempt to provide a more differentiated response to cases. In this respect, it was perhaps the most contentious and sensitive element of *New Directions*, particularly if it was subsequently established that the Department had failed to protect a child because the referral had been inappropriately classified as CCR instead of CMA.

- An increased emphasis on the child in a *family-focused approach* to working with families in the planning and provision of supportive and empowering services.

- A *new description of child maltreatment* which placed greater emphasis on the *harm* experienced by a child rather than on the nature of the act or incident in isolation.

- *Abolition of the category "not substantiated child at risk"*, but an increased recognition of the presence of risk factors in assessment and case management.

- An increased consideration of *the cultural context of referrals*—particularly with Aboriginal families.

- The introduction of a new classification of *priority response times* for CMAs and CCRs. When a referral had been classified and it had been determined that the Department should respond, a decision had to be made as to the time frame for response. *CCRs could be given Priority 1, 2 or 3 status while CMAs could be given only Priority 1 or 2 status*. The definitions were as follows:

  Priority 1: Where a child is in immediate risk of harm or a current family crisis requires immediate attention to secure the safety of the family and children, a response is required immediately within one working day.

  Priority 2: Where the risk of harm to a child or current family crisis requires a response within two to five working days.

  Priority 3: In relation to CCRs only, where no harmful circumstances are involved, as assessment or response would be commenced within 10 working days.

New Directions was an explicit attempt by the Department to move away from a narrow forensic concern with child maltreatment investigations toward a more differentiated approach, which would also put a greater emphasis on family support and providing services on a voluntary basis to families on the basis of partnership. It is important to note that the use of the categories CMA and CCR depended not only on the nature of the concern and whether there was any evidence of harm or injury to the child, but also on whether the information available suggested that the Department had a mandate to compel cooperation:

A child maltreatment allegation is a referral which suggests that a child has been harmed, or is likely to suffer harm or injury, as opposed to general concerns about a child. One critical difference between CMAs and CCRs was that when dealing with allegations of maltreatment, the department has a clear reason to compel the subject/s of a child protection investigation to cooperate through reference to the powers conferred under legislation.

This is different to dealing with CCRs because, in the absence of any information to suggest that a child may have been or is at risk of harm through maltreatment, the department does not have a reason to compel the family to cooperate with the assessment or accept services.

(Department of Family and Children's Services 1996: 19)

The introduction of *New Directions* had a considerable impact. As Table 3.1 demonstrates, while the total number of official CMA allegations went down dramatically, the substantiation rate went up. The number of CCRs was more than double the number of CMAs. Taken together, the total number or CMAs and CCRs (7,822) in 1998/99 showed a 25 percent increase on the total number or CMAs in 1994/95.

The introduction of *New Directions* made a significant impact on the work of the Western Australian statutory child welfare department. In particular, it helped the department prioritize its work on the basis of a clear rationale. The primary focus became "high risk" cases articulated through a more specific and stringent operational definition of the CMA in a context of continuing high demand (Parton and Mathews 2001). In the process, the way it did this demonstrated some of the major challenges for any department introducing "differential response." CCRs were more likely to be given the lowest priority response time and were less likely to receive non-assessment services. While about a third went on to receive family support services, a similar proportion received the outcome "no viable departmental role." These latter cases were quite likely to be referred again within a year, and contributed to the high overall proportion of CCRs (27 percent) that repeated as a CCR or CMA (Parton and Mathews 2001). Also, Aboriginal families were disproportionately represented in the CCR population such that the CCR classification appeared

Table 3.1 Child maltreatment allegations and substantiations and CCRs 1994/95–1998/99

Financial year	Total allegations	Total substantiations	Substantiation rate (%)	Total CCRs
1994/95	6,237	1,430	24.3	–
1995/96	3,720	1,050	29.9	2,539
1996/97	2,099	982	52.3	5,793
1997/98	2,452	1,136	50.2	5,782
1998/99	2,535	1,166	49.4	5,287

Source: Parton and Mathews 2001: 111

to legitimize less, or no, provision of services for many Aboriginal children and their families. This was also a major issue for concerns about neglect more generally.

It is unsurprising that, following a protracted media frenzy associated with the coronial inquest into the tragic death of a child known to the department in Western Australia, similar changes to those described in other jurisdictions and countries have subsequently occurred. As a result of media pressure, an inquiry was instigated and it recommended a major organizational split into a dedicated and highly forensic Department of Child Protection and a separate Department for Communities (Ford 2007). Simultaneously, albeit though this was not a recommendation of this Report, and as a result of relentless pressure from the political opposition and disturbing reports about child sexual abuse in Indigenous communities, mandatory reporting of child sexual abuse by three professional groups—police, medical practitioners and nurses—was introduced (Children and Community Services Amendment [Reporting Sexual Abuse of Children] Bill 2007).

While evaluations of "differential response" models in the US (for example, US Department of Health and Human Services 2003; Daro *et al.* 2005; Johnson *et al.* 2005; Loman and Siegel 2005; Sawyer and Lohrbach 2005; Shusterman *et al.* 2005; Waldfogel 2008) are more positive, there is a clear danger that all that is achieved is a reshuffling of cases into different categories in order to work within limited resources, rather than working to reduce the incidence of child abuse and neglect (McCallum and Eades 2001).

Integrating "child protection" and "family support"

While we can see the "refocusing debate" in England, following the *Audit Commission report* (1994) and *Child Protection: Messages from Research* (Department of Health 1995), as attempting to introduce a "differential response," its aims were much more ambitious. It attempted to provide an *integrated* approach, which aimed to bring together the major elements of both child protection *and* family support. In the light of the research reviewed, *Messages from Research* (Department of Health 1995) made a number of suggestions as to how "children's safety" could be improved. It emphasized:

- the importance of sensitive and informed professional–client relationships, where honesty and reliability were valued;
- the need for an appropriate balance of power between participants where serious attempts were made to work in partnership;
- a wide perspective on child protection, concerned not only with investigating forensic evidence but also with notions of welfare, prevention and treatment;
- that priority should be afforded to effective supervision and the training of social workers;

- that, generally, the most effective protection from abuse was brought about by "enhancing children's quality of life."

More specifically, it called for a "rebalancing" of child protection work which prioritized Section 17 and Part 3 of the Children Act 1989 in terms of supporting families with "children in need," and thereby keeping notions of policing and coercive intervention to a minimum. It similarly suggested that Section 47 of the Act should be understood as a duty to *enquire*, rather than simply a forensically determined power to investigate.

These conclusions had been spelt out in more detail the year before in a paper by Wendy Rose (1994), in which she shared some of the thinking within the Department of Health on the relationship between child protection and family support and the intentions of the Children's Act 1989. There were two themes which provided the core of her argument. First, she felt that current practices tended to polarize family support and child protection services as distinct and even contrasting activities. She argued that "we should be promoting *one integrated approach* to the local authority's duties under Part 3 and Part 5 of the Act" (Rose 1994: 5, emphasis added). Second, she questioned whether the balance between investigation/assessment processes and the provision of support services best served "children in need." The goal was an *integrated* child care system that encompassed both family support and treatment services and that *rebalanced* child welfare and child protection.

However, the then Conservative government did not take a strong lead in attempts to "refocus" children's services; this was seen as the responsibility of local authorities and very few extra resources were provided. It was clear that local authorities were struggling to respond positively. Research evaluating the Children Act 1989 (Department of Health 2001) in the period leading up to the election of the New Labour government in May 1997 demonstrated that, while there was some evidence of a response to the "refocusing" initiative, a preoccupation with "risk" still dominated intervention at the point of intake. It seemed that in the initial screening of families, the identification of the risk of child abuse continued to be the key criterion for accessing resources (Brandon *et al.* 1999; Thoburn *et al.* 2000; Tunstill and Aldgate 2000). Jane Aldgate summarized the situation as follows:

> The conclusions from the research which has evaluated the implementation of Section 17 over the first eight or so years, suggest that progress has not been straightforward. The Children Act was implemented at a time when investigation of child abuse dominated practice. The concept of identifying children in need based on the impact of impairment or harm was some distance away from an approach which was focusing on identifying risk and the commission of abuse and neglect. With hindsight, the aim of allowing social services and other agencies to identify children in need and set local priorities for service provision was too complex for the primitive technical infrastructure of the time. It was also

difficult to shift the attitudes of local authorities to the broader perspective of family support.

(Aldgate 2002: 164–5)

It seems that the balance between child protection and family support was not being achieved and, more particularly, families who required help where children were "in need" for reasons other than "child maltreatment" were not always gaining access to services. The research studies revealed the need for a more discriminatory matching of children's needs to services, and planning to be linked to welfare outcomes for *all* children in need (Statham and Aldgate 2003).

If "refocusing" and greater "integration" were to be achieved, the research indicated there was a "need for a wider system of assessment that could lead to differential and well-planned patterns of intervention" (Department of Health 2001: 46). For these issues to be addressed, a quite new role for the central state was required, for it seemed clear that local authorities, left to their own initiative, were unable to do so in any consistent and coherent way. With the election of the New Labour government in May 1997 this was about to change.

What became clear soon after New Labour came into power was that the government was keen to broaden the "refocusing initiative" beyond simply rebalancing child protection and family support, to embrace wide-ranging concerns about parenting, the need for early intervention to tackle crime and antisocial behavior, supporting the family, and regenerating communities more generally. This was to become a key responsibility for local authorities generally, rather than just social service departments, and was to reposition the role of health, education and criminal justice agencies as well as the non-government sector, and where the development of early years services was to be given priority. In essence, concerns about the state of children, childhood, and parenting more generally were to be the subject of a whole series of government policies and initiatives, and it was the Home Office and the Treasury, as well as the Department of Health, which were to take the lead. Paul Boateng, then Parliamentary Undersecretary of State for Health, gave an indication of future policy at a conference in March 1998:

This government is committed to ensuring we support families, especially in their parenting role, so as to give children the best start in life. We are committed to supporting families when they seek help, and before they reach crisis point, and to making the best use of scarce public resources. It is because of that we see the importance of early intervention. The evidence is that early intervention works.

(Boating 1999: 14)

From the outset, New Labour had a much wider and more proactive approach to policies toward children than simply protecting children from abuse. Such policies lay at the core of its attempts to refashion the welfare state. Childhood moved to the center of policy because it was seen as being at the fulcrum of New Labour attempts to tackle social exclusion and invest in a positive and wealth-creating knowledge economy (Parton 2006a,b).

The impact of this new approach was made clear with the publication of the new government guidance on child protection. Whereas the 1991 version, published to coincide with the implementation of the 1989 Children Act, was entitled *Working Together under the Children Act 1989: A Guide to Arrangements for Inter-agency Co-operation for the Protection of Children from Abuse* (Home Office *et al.* 1991), by 1999 it had become *Working Together to Safeguard Children: A Guide to Inter-agency Working to Safeguard and Promote the Welfare of Children* (Department of Health *et al.* 1999). The focus had broadened from "the protection of children from abuse" to "safeguarding and promoting the welfare of children." The document was a clear reflection of the need not just to refocus child protection and family support but to locate such work in New Labour's broader agendas in relation to children and parents. For this to happen it was clear a more rigorous, integrated and overarching approach to assessment was required, and the publication of the 1999 edition of *Working Together* was combined with the publication of the *Framework for the Assessment of Children in Need and their Families* (Department of Health *et al.* 2000). The "Assessment Framework" was an explicit attempt to move practice, which was almost exclusively concerned with the risk of significant harm to the child, to an approach which aimed to identify impairment in the context of children's development—both safeguarding and promoting children's welfare—and where the focus was a child's "needs." As Jenny Gray, who had the lead responsibility for developing the "Assessment Framework" at the Department of Health, argued, the "Framework":

> was developed on the understanding that assessing whether a child is in need and identifying the nature of this need requires a systematic approach which uses the same framework or conceptual map to gather and analyse information about all children and their families, but discriminates effectively between different types and levels of need.
>
> (Gray 2002: 176)

However, if there was any doubt about the significance of these developments, the challenges involved, and the complexities which practitioners were expected to address, these were quickly dispelled. For, just as the new *Working Together* and the "Assessment Framework" were being introduced in 2000, the public inquiry into the tragic death of Victoria Climbié was announced. At the core of the inquiry was a major concern about how the case had been categorized for the purposes of assessment and intervention by the various agencies involved. Specifically, the inquiry report strongly argued that the case was defined as a "child in need," as opposed to a "child protection" case, and was taken less seriously as a result. This was seen as a major factor contributing to her death and the report argued that prioritizing work in this way was quite unacceptable. If a "child in need" was responded to inadequately, particularly if this was done in an unfocused, unsystematic and uncoordinated way, the implications for all the professionals concerned were no different than if the case had been treated as a child protection investigation.

> It is not possible to separate the protection of children from wider support to families. Indeed, often the best protection for a child is achieved by the timely intervention of family support services. The wholly unsatisfactory practice, demonstrated so often in the Inquiry, of determining the needs of a child before an assessment has been completed, reinforces in me the belief that "referrals" should not be labelled "child protection" without good reason. The needs of the child and his or her family are often inseparable.
>
> (Laming Report 2003, para 1.30)

And perhaps more forcibly:

> The single most important change in the future must be the drawing of a clear line of accountability from the top to the bottom without doubt or ambiguity about who is responsible at every level for the *well-being of vulnerable children.*
>
> (*Ibid.*, para 1.2, emphasis added)

By the early years of the new millennium it was clear that simply trying to differentiate cases was not seen as good enough, nor was responding with a forensically determined child protection investigation as previously. What was needed was an integrated approach which attempted to improve the "well-being of vulnerable children."

Improving the "well-being" of children

We can identify a number of themes and trends which are evident across the jurisdictions. Whether, and how far, these have been developed is enormously variable, let alone whether they are being successful. Even so, we can see a general attempt to move the focus of policy and practice away from a narrow focus on child protection to one which is much more concerned with early intervention and the improvement of children's "well-being." Adam Tomison (2004) has provided a useful resumé of these developments and suggests a number of "service trends" have become evident over recent years:

*   crisis services addressing issues such as family violence, have increasingly been complemented by services that build on family strengths (capacity-building) and the creation of resiliency using a solution-focused approach;

- family support services try to take account of wider structural or community-level factors that might impact on service delivery, such as poverty, social isolation and a lack of key support services;
- an increased investment in early childhood and early intervention programs, which emphasize the importance of a positive environment for children's development, particularly in the first three years of life;
- an increased focus on service integration, inter-agency coordination and the development of cross-sectoral responses to a range of problems affecting children and young children, including child maltreatment;
- encouraging the voluntary engagement of "at risk" families, where the concerns related to children are not considered serious enough to warrant statutory action, to seek out and use family support services;
- a focus on the creation of flexible, innovative service solutions that are locally designed and tailored to meet the needs of specific communities, including Indigenous, rural and remote communities;
- a growing recognition that family support services should address the needs of all family members including mothers, fathers, children and key members of extended families; and
- a greater focus on measuring outcomes and evaluating program impact in order to develop and implement an evidence-based approach to policy and practice.

Such developments are particularly evident in England. The publication of the Green Paper *Every Child Matters* (Chief Secretary to the Treasury 2003) and the passage of the Children Act 2004 marked a significant shift in thinking about children's services in England and heralded a major period of reform and change (Department for Education and Skills 2004; HM Government 2005). The pace and nature of change in England seems of a different order to elsewhere, and is related to attempts to "modernize" services and practices, in the context of the major social changes of the previous 30 years (Parton 2006a,b).

While the changes were presented as a direct response to the public inquiry into the death of Victoria Climbié, they were much more than this. They aimed to ensure that "every child" fulfilled their potential. The changes take forward the idea that it is important to intervene in children's lives at an early stage in order to prevent problems later in life, particularly in relation to educational attainment, unemployment, crime and social exclusion more generally. They build on much of the research and thinking that had become evident by the mid 1990s, and which formed the basis of many of the policies introduced by the New Labour government after 1997 in relation to children and childhood, where child development was seen as key and where children were conceptualized as future citizens requiring both safeguarding and investment (Hendrick 2003; Fawcett *et al.* 2004; Featherstone 2006). The combination of wanting to introduce changes, which would both broaden the scope of prevention while trying to reduce the chances of a child dying in the tragic circumstances experienced by Victoria Climbié, meant that the role of the state would become broader, more interventive and regulatory at the same time. In the words of the then Minister for Children, Young People and Families, in her foreword to *Every Child Matters: Next Steps* (Department for Education and Skills 2004), the vision is of "a shift to prevention while strengthening protection" (p. 3). The overall aim of the changes is to improve the "well-being" of all children according to five outcomes:

- *Be healthy*: enjoying good physical and mental health and living a healthy lifestyle.
- *Stay safe*: being protected from harm and abuse.
- *Enjoy and achieve*: getting the most out of life and developing the skills for adulthood.
- *Making a positive contribution*: being involved with the community and society and not engaging in anti-social or offending behavior; and
- *Achieve economic well-being*: not being prevented by economic disadvantage from achieving their full potential.

Every Child Matters: Change for Children (HM Government 2005) provides the national framework for local change programs in England, led by local authorities, including an "outcomes framework" against which changes at the local level will be judged and inspected. Each of the overall outcomes has five aims, and "staying safe" has just one of its aims as "safe from maltreatment, neglect, violence and sexual exploitation," which has as its primary "indicator" "re-registration on the child protection register." Concerns about "maltreatment" are just a small element of this ambitious program of change for children. What is clear is that the government has created a managerialized framework for both promoting and assessing children's development, with an audit system of targets and performance indicators. Responsibility for achieving the targets, however, resides primarily with parents together with a range of health, welfare and criminal justice professionals, in the newly reconfigured children's services, who will support, monitor, and enforce parents', children's and young people's behaviors.

Underpinning the changes are two assumptions concerning the nature of contemporary social life and the state of current knowledge. First, the Green Paper (HM Government 2005) stated that, over the previous generation, children's lives had undergone "profound change." While children now had more opportunities than ever before and had generally benefited from rising prosperity and better health, they also faced more uncertainties and risks. They faced earlier exposure to sexual activity, drugs, and alcohol, and family patterns had changed significantly. There were more lone parents, more divorces, and more women in paid employment, all of which had made family life more complex and, potentially, made the position of children more precarious.

Second, however, the Green Paper asserted that these changes had come about at a time when we now had increased knowledge and expertise and, therefore, were in a better position to respond to these new uncertainties and risks. In particular, "we better understand the importance of early influences on the development of values and behaviour" (HM Government 2005: 15). It was thus important to ensure that this knowledge was drawn upon to inform the changes being introduced. For "we have a good idea what factors shape children's life chances. Research tells us that the risk of experiencing negative outcomes is concentrated in children with certain characteristics and experiences" (HM Government 2005: 17).

While research had not built up a detailed picture of the causal links, certain factors were said to be associated with poor outcomes, and these included:

• low income and parental unemployment
• homelessness
• poor parenting
• poor schooling
• postnatal depression among mothers
• low birth weight
• substance misuse
• individual characteristics, such as intelligence, and community factors, such as living in a disadvantaged neighborhood.

The more risk factors a child experienced, such as being excluded from school and family breakdown, the more likely it was that they would experience negative outcomes, and the Green Paper argued that:

> research suggests that parenting appears to be the most important factor associated with educational attainment at age ten, which in turn is strongly associated with achievement later in life. Parental involvement in education seems to be a more important influence than poverty, school environment and the influence of peers.
>
> (HM Government 2005: 18)

Because of this increased knowledge about risk factors associated with child development, it was seen as important to intervene at an earlier stage in order to forestall problems in later life. Early intervention in childhood was seen to provide a major strategy for overcoming social exclusion, both for children and for avoiding problems later. While prompted by the Laming Report (2003) into the death of Victoria Climbié, the Green Paper is only tangentially concerned with child abuse. Having asserted that "child protection cannot be separated from policies to improve children's lives as a whole" (para.4), the Green Paper then set out a framework for "protective" services to cover all children and young people from birth to 19, the aim of which is to "reduce the numbers of children who experience educational failure, engage in offending or antisocial behavior, suffer from ill-health, or become teenage parents" (para.4).

The other area where it is asserted that knowledge and expertise had grown and which was seen as vital in order to take policy and practice forward, was in relation to the major developments in information and communication technology (ICT). The age of electronic government was seen as having major implications for the reform and development of children's services. Not only would this provide the potential for identifying problems and enhancing attempts to intervene at an earlier stage, but it would also allow different organizations and professionals to share information in order to ensure that children's problems were not missed and, crucially, children did not fall through "the net." The introduction of more integrated services was seen as crucially dependent on the introduction of new ICT. Three key developments aimed to take this forward.

First, *ContactPoint*, previously the *Information Sharing Index* (IS Index). Section 12 of the Children Act 2004 requires children's services authorities to establish databases on *all children* living in the area served by the authority. The databases are not intended to be narrowly focused on child protection but aim to improve the sharing of information between professionals, in order to improve the well-being of *all children*, in terms of the five broad outcomes. The information will comprise: name; address; date of birth; a unique identifying number; name and contact details of any person with parental responsibility or who has day-to-day care of the child; details of any education being received whether in an education institution or other setting; and the name and contact details of the general practitioner. Originally there was also the provision for the inclusion of name and contact details of any practitioner providing a specialist service, and that the practitioner had "a cause for concern." The draft regulations identified three areas where extra information should be included on the database; where a named professional (a) considered that s/he has important information to share relating to the person; or (b) had undertaken an assessment of the person under the system known as the *Common Assessment Framework* (CAF) (see below); or, (c) has taken action relating to the person. No material relating to an individual or family would be included on the database, so that it would be up to any practitioner accessing the database to contact whoever flagged the "cause for concern" to find out further details.

From the beginning major criticisms were voiced about the database including that its introduction suggested, for the first time, England would have a form of a mandatory reporting system (Munro and Parton 2007). In May 2007 the information system was rebranded as *ContactPoint* and the criteria whereby professionals would place an "indication" of concern on the database were modified. Then, in November 2007, it was announced, in the light of massive security leaks with other government confidential databases, that the introduction of *ContactPoint* was to be put back even further and subject to further review. It is very unclear at the time of writing whether it will be introduced and, if it is, in what format. Considerable concerns have been raised about the security of the database, its implications for the civil liberties and human rights of both children and parents, and the general utility and cost-effectiveness of the scheme (Parton 2008).

Second, the CAF is an electronic assessment form to be completed by any professional when they consider that a child might have "additional needs" that require the involvement of more than one service. The idea is that it will save time as one assessment can be used thereafter. It includes a wide-ranging set of data covering most aspects of a child's health and development, including details about the parents and siblings. It follows the format introduced by the "Assessment Framework."

Third, the *Integrated Children's System* (ICS) is designed for children's social services and will include the case records and details of all children and families known to social workers whether they are in "care", on the child protection register or a "child in need." The extent to which this information might also be linked to related electronic information systems in health, education and criminal justice is not yet clear.

Taken together, the changes currently being introduced are the most radical anywhere in the Anglophone world. England is in the process of introducing what one of us has called previously (Parton 2008) "the preventive-surveillance state," which aims to intervene earlier rather than simply respond to crises, but which also poses direct and indirect threats to civil liberties and human rights via its wide-ranging and detailed systems of surveillance and information sharing.

Managerialization and proceduralization

While such an approach can be seen to be attempting to move well beyond previous policy initiatives to provide a "differential response," "refocus," or "integrate," it can also be seen to epitomize many of the characteristics of child protection policy and practice over the last 30 years. For attempts to "reform" child protection and child welfare more generally have been dominated by managerialist approaches which put ever greater emphasis upon intro-ducing sophisticated systems, procedures, assessment, demands and "outcome frameworks." The period has seen the increased curtailment of professional discretion and the requirement that front-line professionals follow increasingly detailed and complex procedural guidance. This has grown considerably with the increasing use of computers and various ICT systems, and where the gathering, sifting, assessment, sharing, and monitoring of information (Parton 2007) has become central. Ironically, attempts in England to move policy and practice away from an emphasis upon a narrow, forensic and investi-gatory approach have had the effect of increasing the managerialization and proceduralization of the work even further and, in the process, has included a wider range of children, parents, and professionals in the orbit of surveillance.

The collection, classifying and management of information have taken on a strategic significance for both safeguarding *and* promoting the welfare of children, and holding professionals to account. Thus, while the amount of "technicality" in the work has increased, the amount of "indeterminacy" has decreased and the work has become managerialized:

> The rise of the manager in social work sees the introduction of a range of skills related largely to defining and measuring performance and outcome. Such an outlook seeks to establish routines, standardize practices and predictable task environments. It is antithetical to depth explanations, professional discretion, creative practice, and tolerance of complexity and uncertainty.
>
> (Howe 1996: 92)

In suggesting that the focus has become measuring performance and outcomes, we need to recognize that this not only applies to social work practitioners but those with whom they work—particularly children, young people, and their parents and carers, and other professionals.

As Carol Smith (2001) has argued, the situation is full of paradox, for while most agree that certainty is not possible, the political and organizational climate demands it. Social workers have been found wanting and are no longer trusted. The result is that many of the changes introduced act to sidestep the paradox and substitute *confidence in systems* for *trust in individual professionals*, so that the introduction of the most up-to-date technology becomes the key element for judging and managing change. The continual refinement and reform of "systems" demonstrate that services for children are conceived, increasingly, as instrumental machines which need to be updated to take account of new challenges and the new knowledges and technologies that are available. The fact that they may have failed points only to the need for their repair, and new procedures, diagrams and flow charts are required to make the increased complexity of the systems comprehensible. The emphasis on coordination and the management and sharing of information testifies to the complexity of the organizational environment in which the work takes place.

Within these new governmental strategies for children's services, audit has become one of the key mechanisms for responding to failure, the most dramatic and high profile being the regular use of the public inquiry. According to Michael Power (1994, 1997) audit and inspection have come to replace the trust once accorded to professionals. Audit responds to the failure and insecurity by the managerialization of risk. Risk is rendered manageable by new relations of regulation between the political centers of decision making and the front-line professionals, via the introduction of a variety of procedures, forms, and systems for making and noting decisions, and thereby making them visible. In the process, the professionals and the people with whom they work are transformed in order to make them both auditable and responsible. Where the key concern is risk, the priority is liable to be making a *defensive* decision where the required procedures have been followed rather than making the *right* decision (Dingwall *et al.* 1995; Parton 1996). The danger is that, in an area of work which is highly sensitive and where the media are always looking for "mistakes" so that any case is potentially high profile, trust is difficult to maintain. Such developments have generated systems which are relatively closed to the possibility of relationship-based practice, and which fail to recognize the importance of negotiation, mediation, and professional judgment, and the crucial need to develop trust.

> Trust at its most fundamental level involves a belief by the population that the state is basically benign, and that state services are essentially there for their benefit. This is notwithstanding the conflicts of interest which will inevitably emerge in welfare delivery. The state in turn must trust the families to bring up their children, and must be driven by the basic belief that families who need help are entitled to support by right, rather than that these families are failures in need of surveillance and monitoring. The state and the community should also feel able to trust professionals to exercise their professional judgement to assess or intervene when necessary and to ensure the fair and equitable distribution of resources.
>
> (Cooper *et al.* 2003: 31)

At the core of these problems is what Cooper *et al.* call a "confidentiality crisis" (Cooper *et al.* 2003: 15). For while, on the one hand, confidentiality is deemed to be a fundamental part of the professional–client relationship and is essential if the relationship is to be built on trust, on the other hand, professionals are required to share information not only to aid child protection but also, in England, to ensure that all children reach their potential (Munro and Parton 2007). Clients become sources of information so that assessments can be made, resources allocated and the child's development monitored.

While the trends and developments in policy and practice identified by Tomison (2004), summarized earlier, have many positive dimensions to them, the overall culture in which they are located is not consistent with the values and practices which are likely to have positive outcomes. The dominance of a managerialist, audit culture fails to recognize the centrality of trust and the nature of the complexities involved. It fails to recognize the key relational aspects to the work and what children, young people, parents, and carers say they most value. The key to improving policy and practice resides in recognizing the crucial ethical and moral dimensions to the work and that reform which concentrates on technical systems reform is quite inadequate. We shall return to this in the following chapters, but first will attend to a factor that is currently contributing to the serious pressures confronting child protection agencies in most, but not all, jurisdictions—the escalation of child protection reports and its effects on system responses and outcomes.

Workload and service delivery outcomes

While differential response was an important initiative taken to respond to rising workload demands and limited resources, it has not been entirely successful in this regard, with evidence in a number of jurisdictions of continuing escalating demand, sometimes making it very difficult for front-line staff to keep up (Shireman 2003; Mansell 2006a,b; D. Scott 2006b). For example, between 1999 and 2005 the number of reports (notifications) to Australian child protection authorities doubled, with the numbers in New South Wales witnessing a 246 percent increase (E. Scott 2006). Reports have risen for a variety of complex and interrelated reasons, including:

• the general public becoming more aware of abuse and neglect and demanding an increased level of risk assurance (Mansell 2006b);
• changes in legislation, policy and practices that have contributed to net-widening by expanding definitional criteria and thereby including low-risk matters for investigation follow up (Mansell 2006a,b; D. Scott 2006a; E. Scott 2006; Pelton 2008);
• child protection agencies' internal processes for handling reports, which can hinder reliable and timely feedback to the staff regarding the accuracy of their interpretations and decision making about the need for investigation responses (Mansell 2006a,b);
• mandatory reporting and inclusion of domestic violence matters that police have attended (E. Scott 2006; Pelton 2008);
• increased media attention, particularly following scandals, which influences an anxious public to report and a risk-averse staff to interpret and define events as "at risk" and to be investigated, rather than make a mistake (Mansell 2006a); and
• in many jurisdictions, the only way to access services is via the child protection system, thereby forcing people to seek help by reporting the matter to statutory authorities (Pelton 2008).

Mansell's (2006a,b) research of the factors affecting demand in New Zealand has been important in shedding light onto the complexity of issues affecting organizational processes and responses to changes in demand, and the difficulties confronting staff in trying to deal with increased community insistence for satisfactory risk assurance about the safety and well-being of children. There are often very limited options for containing demand within the existing resource and organizational capacity to deal with it, and Mansell argues that differential response and other typical strategies will only have a limited impact given the nature of contemporary child protection systems and the conflicting community demands. He concludes that:

> One solution might be to seek to rebalance the government response to children in need by moving resources toward a general child welfare model

and reducing the more forensic, statutory child protection response . . . again, as mere policy dictate this is unlikely to work, unless it also changes the underlying system dynamics that will demand increased responsiveness over time. Without changing the system dynamics, such solutions will tend over time to unravel and revert to a forensic emergency response (child protection).

(Mansell 2006a: 92)

We agree with Mansell that more is needed than just altering definitional criteria and that reform of some of the fundamental aspects of contemporary approaches and structures is needed. This is not to suggest that all is bad with the current systems, or that child protection approaches are not appropriate and necessary in many situations. Rather, we believe that applying what is largely a forensic approach to all cases deemed "at risk" is counterproductive and is not producing the outcomes for service users that a civil society expects.

In the following chapters we will focus on what is not working well in current systems and make a case for their reform. However, it needs to be emphasized that there is considerable diversity across and within Anglophone countries regarding systems and their outcomes, and there are many positive signs and significant successes regarding children's safety and well-being. For example, the USA is quite different from other countries with regard to levels of violent crime, and access to weapons and drugs. In a recent article, David Finkelhor and Lisa Jones (2006) examined a range of child maltreatment and victimization data from the USA since the early 1990s and explored the reasons for declines in a number of areas, albeit with neglect rates increasing. These overall trends are welcome news indeed. However, the article did not address the outcomes for service users, particularly children in care and parents, nor the issues surrounding the levels of reports of abuse and neglect, and the implications of increased social surveillance, which we argue are also important characteristics of any social care and social control system. Furthermore, there was little detailed examination of sociological factors such as the welfare-to-work reforms, social angst against paedophilia and child abuse scandals, and the influence of a risk society that is more ready to surveil and punish. Nevertheless, their conclusion that the "the era of continually rising numbers of child maltreatment and crime victimization cases is probably over" (Finkelhor and Jones 2006: 709) is strongly positive for children and young people, and also with regard to the implications for the role of child protection systems. Signs of reducing victimization are encouraging. In the following chapters we examine the broad systemic outcomes of child protection systems in Anglophone countries, with a particular focus on the organizational environments, and the experiences of service users, staff, and community stakeholders.

4 The troubled state of organizational environments

We have outlined how a social movement based upon a broad community mandate expressing concern for children and families and their well-being has developed over time to be called "child protection," and the manner in which the underlying ideologies and values have altered to produce and shape the social institutions and professional practice established to respond to these anxieties (Ferguson 2004; Merrick 2006). We now turn to critically examine the nature of the structures, cultures, processes and practices of the organizations given the difficult tasks of surveilling the population, particularly those sections considered "dangerous," and intervening to ensure the safety and well-being of children deemed vulnerable to child abuse and neglect—those "at risk."

In this examination we highlight the key themes that have emerged, which demonstrate that these systems are failing in their assigned tasks—their "missions" in contemporary management parlance. We will identify the interconnected reasons for understanding why these organizations have often become "toxic" environments for those who govern and manage them, and work in them to set and implement policy, and for the multiplicity of children, families and communities they profess to serve (Glisson and Hemmelgarn 1998; Aronson and Sammon 2000; Dollard *et al.* 2001; Mor Barak *et al.* 2001; Bednar 2003; Smith 2005; Wells 2006; Pelton 2008). Contemporary organizations are diverse, complex and dynamic in their processes and operations and it is not our intention to suggest that they are the same everywhere. Rather, we posit that despite their different contexts and locations within a variety of social and community contexts, there are a number of identifiable themes evident in the ways that they do their business, and that statutory child protection agencies are typified by their mission failures rather than their successes. In fact, these failures have often provided the basis and drive for significant change. Yet, despite innumerable valiant attempts to restructure and reform them, the available evidence overwhelmingly indicates that they are failing and have been for some time. As the key tool for enacting the broad social mandate, child protection systems are unsustainable in their current form.

Organizational failure

Nowadays, all organizations (be they government or non-government) are expected to be efficient and high performing, and strategic management is often used as a proactive process of analytical thinking and action to promote growth and development. Organizational restructuring is one method employed to reduce costs and ensure continued relevance to changed operational contexts, albeit within the current dominant management discourse (Hirsch and De Soucey 2006). However, within this perspective there is an assumption that inefficient and ineffective organizations cease to operate, which research has found is not always the case, particularly in contexts where there are numerous competing stakeholders and contested organizational missions (Meyer and Zucker 1989).

We contend that, notwithstanding contextual diversity around the world, generally speaking, child protection organizations and systems are characterized by failure to achieve their complex and contested mission—protecting all children from harm and ensuring their ongoing safety. The reasons for their failure are complex, but essentially the "core business" has gradually been expanded over time due to pressures from a multiplicity of stakeholders, with significant dispute concerning what exactly the social mandate and functions of these agencies should be, who their central clientele are (Children? Parents? Community?), what their modus operandi should entail (investigation/assessment/treatment/prevention?), and what their key goals, outcomes and performance indicators are (the "deliverables"). Given the politicized nature of their existence, these organizations and their ways of operating are now so hotly contested as to be virtually unachievable to the satisfaction of anyone.

Further, they are incapable of fundamental reforms without substantial alteration to their central mission and resources to enable their transformation and reform. In essence, the original mission of promoting child welfare and preventing abuse and neglect has been broadened to the point of excluding little by way of harm to children, with child protection organizations being given a remit that is unattainable and unsustainable. Moreover, with their mission, goals, and practice approaches contested among a variety of dependent actors (Mildred 2003), their actions and achievements are usually subject to considerable criticism, which is often couched in the language of "accountability," but is nevertheless tantamount to a pervasive "blame culture" that affects all the dependent actors (Parton 1996; Holland and Scourfield 2004; Munro 2004b).

Systemically speaking, the "outcome" realities of child protection organizations include the following:

- While protecting many children from abuse and neglect, they are also prone to unacceptable levels of false positives and false negatives (Munro 1999a).

- The social, economic and other costs upon families of catch-all risk management approaches to reports are significant, but are not necessarily included in organizational, policy and practice considerations (Johnson and Petrie 2004; Munro 2004a; Pelton 2008).
- They are generally incapable of providing the necessary assistance and resources to families to prevent further abuse and neglect occurring because of a preoccupation with surveillance and investigation (Cooper *et al.* 2003; Shireman 2003; D. Scott 2006a; Pelton 2008).
- Taken overall, the negative life experiences and outcomes of children who are in care (e.g. offending, low educational attainment etc), particularly for those who have many placements, are appalling, leading to serious questioning of the fostering system (Gilbertson and Barber 2003, 2004; Pecora *et al.* 2003, 2005, 2006; Shireman 2003; Mendes 2005; Courtney and Dworsky 2006; Stein 2006; Wade and Dixon 2006; Berridge 2007).
- The huge personal costs on staff including significant work stress, burnout, vicarious trauma and associated job dissatisfaction (Anderson 2000; Aronson and Sammon 2000; McLean and Andrew 2000; Dollard *et al.* 2001; Mor Barak *et al.* 2001; Bednar 2003; Morris 2005; Weaver *et al.* 2007).
- The financial costs of running the system continue to escalate while their performance steadily declines (Ainsworth and Hansen 2006; E. Scott 2006; Mansell 2006a,b).

Despite such clear evidence of their ineffectiveness and poor performance, which is tantamount to gross organizational failure, it is "business as usual", albeit within a context of repeated structural reorganizations and policy alterations. There are sometimes significant reforms, such as differential response measures in the USA (Waldfogel 1998, 2008) and the *Every Child Matters* program in England (Parton 2006b), which have entailed major changes to policy and practice, but with little overall success in the outcomes achieved vis-à-vis the safety and well-being of children and families. We will now examine the influential factors and processes that have contributed to this situation, review key indicators of organizational performance, and identify the reasons for their failures.

Ideology and the reconstructed welfare state

In Chapter 3 we touched upon the managerialization and proceduralization of child protection practice as a result of regular attempts to reform the system. These processes, however, did not occur in a vacuum but were part of a far broader reform agenda for the public sector, particularly in Anglophone countries (Harris 1998; Aronson and Sammon 2000; McDonald *et al.* 2003; Argy 2004; Abramovitz 2005; Meuller and Carter 2005; Mitchell *et al.* 2005; McDonald 2006). Moreover, the reforms struck at the very fundamentals of the welfare state, in what Gilbert (2002) has suggested was the silent surrender of public responsibility.

It is debatable where precisely the push for reform of the state and welfare began, but it undoubtedly had much of its intellectual push from resurgent neoclassical economists and the significant alterations to the post-war fiscal arrangements affecting finance, trade and production economics (McDonald 2006). Western capitalist economies were placed under considerable pressure as a result of events such as the breakdown of fixed exchange rates, an increasingly global world market, deindustrialization and the advent of post-Fordist production methods, and resultant economic and social regulation (McDonald 2006; Jordan 2006, 2007). This occurred with the geopolitical backdrop of the Cold War, the rise of political, economic and military power of the USA, and the advent of the European Union in what was a period of significant global tensions and conflicts.

A period of rapid social, economic and technological change occurred during the latter half of the twentieth century. Many developed industrialized economies experienced hard times including high unemployment and inflation, with significant periods of low or negative economic growth (Jordan 2006, 2007). With economic policy increasingly predominant among political considerations and largely driving social policy, neoconservative politicians gained power in many of the major Western nations and implemented a raft of policy changes that have had profound effects on the role of the state. With market-based economics being embraced as the remedy to economic rejuvenation, large government was seen as antithetical to an efficient and effective economy and prosperity (McDonald 2006). In many countries, but not all, the welfare state was increasingly seen as part of the problem rather than part of the solution, the prescription being a rewriting of the social contract between government and the broad population (Jordan 2006, 2007). There seems little doubt that, generally speaking, we now live in a harsher and more punitive social environment, with the welfare state gradually transformed, and based upon blaming and judgmental social attitudes and residualist policies and services.

There were significant reforms to welfare legislation and child welfare legislation in most Western nations, albeit with very mixed policy agendas and results reported (Aronson and Sammon 2000; Shireman 2003; Shook Slack *et al.* 2003; Farell 2004; Abramovitz 2005; Barton and Welbourne 2005; Mitchell *et al.* 2005; Ashford 2006; Dunifon *et al.* 2006; Pelton 2008). Moreover, social policy is very much a foot servant to economic and labor market policy, a transition that McDonald (2006) calls from "welfare to workfare." The relative power and influence of proponents of social welfare, including the profession of social work, rapidly ebbed away. As McDonald (2006) notes, the "welfare state as an idea, as a set of institutional arrangements and social practices has become increasingly contested, and ultimately, largely discredited in the dominant political debates" (p. 10).

The rise of the neoliberal state entailed five core values: the primacy of individuals rather than collectivist approaches, personal choice as a principle for government, market security, small government, and a *laissez faire* economy (McDonald 2006). Public policies generally embraced privatization and deregulation as central pillars (Argy 2004). Public administrative structures and processes were "reformed" in order to bring about a much more entrepreneurial approach able to promote economic growth, rather than a traditional bureaucratic method. A key part of these reforms of the public sector was the advent and now dominance of "New Public Management" (NPM), often referred to as "Managerialism." Because its impact has been so profound upon the structures and processes currently employed in statutory child protection systems, we will briefly outline its characteristics and critically examine the effects upon child protection policy and practice.

New Public Management

The moves toward "reforming" the public sectors in a range of countries were accompanied by an increasing politicization of its role, function and management (Walter 2006). No longer was elected government to be hamstrung in implementing its policies by bureaucracies that hid behind notions of independence and "the public good" and, arguably, lacked accountability for their outcomes. NPM embraced an array of values, beliefs and practices in its selected mission of "re-engineering" the state and its approach to governance, essentially transforming it via entrepreneurial leadership (McDonald 2006). It is now a dominant ideology that has resulted in management becoming powerful and pre-eminent as a knowledge and skill base, largely supplanting discipline-based professionals as the experts (Harris 1998; Reed 1999; Jones 2001; Tsui and Cheung 2004; Hirsch and De Soucey 2006).

Essentially, it assumes that better management will address any number and range of problems through the application of a regime of tools and processes that provide sophisticated planning, implementation, monitoring, and review of business operations (Tsui and Cheung 2004). This transfer of market-based approaches to the public sector largely occurred without proper consideration of the contextual differences evident between for-profit and government enterprises, various professional groups and discourses, and even among different cultures and states.

A range of tools, techniques and approaches have characterized NPM, including:

- marketization of the provision of welfare services, with splits between government purchasers and not-for-profit and for-profit providers, contractual arrangements, promoting individual choice of service users, increased "user pays" approaches, and strict rationing of scarce resources;

- utilization by executives of strategic management approaches to the development, planning, implementation, monitoring, and review of social policy and programs;
- adopting accountability (internal and external) as a rubric for strong leadership, openness and transparency within decision making and practice;
- an emphasis upon tight control of business operations through strict financial processes and authorizations, and quantifying performance criteria such as targets, outcomes, outputs and inputs, quality assurance, and management;
- reshaping organizational cultures, particularly those of middle managers, to be more in sync with business approaches rather than professional discourses of service orientation, professional standards and addressing the social needs of the disadvantaged;
- embracing human resource management (HRM) and "performance management" as ways to direct and control employees in order to meet organizational objectives and needs;
- utilizing "risk management" strategies and auditing measures across a diverse array of operations; and
- reasserting notions of "partnership" and "community" to foster neoliberal "responsibilization" of citizens at a variety of levels.

There is significant debate about the impact of NPM on a range of public sector systems, institutions and disciplines (Heffernan 2005; Kirkpatrick *et al.* 2005; Bradley and Parker 2006; Diefenbach 2007). Much of this material is critical and NPM's considerable achievements and benefits have been less well recognized, such as greater organizational efficiency and increased flexibility in proactively responding to dynamic economic, social and organizational environments. Notwithstanding these advantages, the literature and research on the impacts on child protection systems are generally portrayed as negative, albeit often with little empirical evidence to establish this (Wells 2006). These managerialist practices in child protection systems have reshaped the relationships between executives, managers and professional staff, with power ebbing away from the latter to the former (Harris 1998; Jones 2001; Cooper *et al.* 2003). A managerialist discourse has gradually dominated over traditional professional discourses, often via the use of performance criteria that reorient what is important in practice and interventions into family life (Froggett 2002) and, second, through the use of accountability measures such as child death reviews and other audit mechanisms (Holland and Scourfield 2004; Munro 2004a; Connolly and Doolan 2006, 2007).

Tilbury (2004, 2005, 2006) has detailed the significant impacts across Anglophone nations that performance measurement has had upon child protection policy and practice including reconceptualizing child abuse and neglect, increased surveillance and accountability but less autonomy for staff, proceduralization, and promotion of a child rescue approach. "Thus, performance measurement has political as well as technical dimensions: it communicates policy intent, shaping the way we think and talk about child protection, defining and redefining notions of outcomes, effectiveness and quality" (Tilbury 2006: 57). It is not surprising that the endless reforms and restructuring of child protection organizations have taken place within a framework of performance measurement of the changes taking place to policy and practice. However, as Wells (2006) notes, there is virtually no empirical evaluative data about how management of child welfare systems affects the outcomes for children.

To implement these measures, the carrot has often been new career opportunities in middle management for professional staff, but the stick has been the threat of punitive consequences for not reaching targets and operating outside policy prescriptions, or worse, decision making resulting in the death of a child. While, by and large, individual casualties among errant professional staff have been rare (public inquiries in the UK being a notable exception), the overall threat perceived by professional staff of public humiliation and career destruction has been pervasive.

The end result has been a rather uneven impact overall, with some professional groups more able than others to resist and renegotiate (Kirkpatrick *et al.* 2005). However, within a weakened welfare state and the human services NPM's impact has been significant (Reed 1999), some suggesting that it was a key tool in restructuring social work culture and practices, making practitioners more like managers and rationers of limited community services (Harris 1998). McDonald (2006) notes that "modern social work draws its primary auspice and moral authority from expressions of the public good, collective responsibility and social justice, notions currently disappearing from the domain of the state as it reshapes itself" (p. 77).

There is little doubt that the overall impact of neoliberal ideologies and NPM has been a fundamental reconstruction of the relationship between the individuals, communities and the state (McDonald 2006; Parton 2006a). The relationships between children, parents, families, and the state have also been reconfigured by the policies and practices adopted within child protection systems (Merrick 2006). As outlined in earlier chapters, this has had a powerful impact because, among other things, services have frequently had an increased social surveillance function, have been targeted at particular groups, and in some countries have adopted a punitive forensic investigatory approach rather than the helping and support orientation common in many European countries.

Case management—part of the problem?

For all its impact on the leadership and administration of the large bureaucracies that statutory child protection systems have become, NPM required a structured mechanism—enhanced accountability measures—to reshape traditional social work and social welfare practice in order to both expose it to managerial oversight, and limit the discretion that individual workers still had in their working relationships with service users. The advent of case management served those purposes well. Moreover, in what was increasingly becoming the "risk society", case management appeared to offer structured processes to undertake risk assessments of complex cases and the auditing of program inputs, outputs, and outcomes. Measuring performance and outcomes directly affects child protection practitioners and those with whom they work.

Initially developed from traditional casework approaches in the human services, case management has become widespread in child protection practice and has been generally viewed as addressing criticisms of social casework. Case management is a more structured and accountable system for the planning, delivery, and coordination of protective interventions and, importantly, emphasizes that services are delivered in accordance with stated policy and procedures. It fitted NPM well as, simultaneously, it has a systemic orientation while also offering an individual focus to service delivery. It replaced casework's emphasis on psychosocially oriented practice with a micro-practice framework that emphasizes client eligibility and responsibilities, staff accountability, and the allocation of limited services and resources to those deemed "high priority" (Froggett 2002).

Case management's flexibility has allowed a number of derivative models, thereby being able to meet the needs of various human service users, organizations, and practitioners with a variety of professional qualifications. Within these system variations there are core processes, including:

- intake;
- assessment;
- case planning and resource identification;
- implementation; and
- monitoring, review, and evaluation.

These processes are congruent with strategic management approaches, particularly assessment, planning, monitoring, and review. The values and beliefs embraced by NPM are also applicable to case management: the approaches to management of an organization are largely replicated in the approach to the management of service users who are given goals and objectives, time frames, and clear outcomes, with close monitoring of progress and a structured review process. Service users are given a clear role in shared decision making, albeit within the boundaries of the "child's best interests." Unfortunately, for most parents, children, and families, this somewhat linearly organized structure has little to do with the reality of implementing change in their lives to overcome the multiple problems and difficulties they experience.

Case management processes have aimed to increase the ability of service users to participate and influence decision making about their lives and the services they receive. While case management structures have sought to engender a greater level of policy and practice congruency, particularly regarding an increased emphasis on collaborative case planning, this often remains dependent upon the discretion afforded to individual case managers. Lipsky's "street level bureaucrats" reminds us that they are the key interpreters, modifiers and implementers of policy into practice (Brodkin 2000; Smith and Donovan 2003; Evans and Harris 2006). However, with the significant deterioration in working relations with service users, particularly with the overt use of power, collaborative decision-making processes can become tokenistic. While many benefits from case management have accrued, including a greater capacity to successfully target services, ascertain service user eligibility and contain program costs, it remains unclear just how these benefits have led to enhanced client outcomes. Further, the approach is no guarantee that sufficient resources will be available and accessible to assist service users. Indeed, there is mounting research evidence that high proportions of identified "at risk" cases are not deemed to be of sufficiently high priority to be allocated resources (Melton and Thompson 2002; Cooper *et al.* 2003; Shireman 2003; Ainsworth and Hansen 2006; D. Scott 2006a; Pelton 2008).

In some jurisdictions, case management systems have embraced "risk assessment" instruments as tools central to the process of determining the nature of the intervention and the level of service delivery required. Proponents have argued that they increase the reliability of assessment decision making and ensure a more consistent level of service, particularly when used by inexperienced staff. Despite claims that empirically based risk assessment instruments are far more reliable and accurate than clinical decision making, they remain controversial in child protection (Gambrill and Shlonsky 2001; Leschied *et al.* 2003; Warner 2003; Shlonsky and Wagner 2005; Pelton 2008). Nevertheless, it is hard to see risk assessment being discarded given the imperative of managing risk in contemporary social work (Stalker 2003; Wells 2006). Within case management systems there are usually detailed policies and guidelines with respect to risk assessment and decision making. Nevertheless, there is considerable uncertainty and ambiguity about where the line must be drawn and how to interpret specific information received in light of these policies (Parton and O'Byrne 2000). Practice wisdom and intuition are important aids to guide workers through these complex assessment processes (Parton and O'Byrne 2000; Munro 2002; Froggett 2002).

As can be seen below, many child protection systems experience high staff turnover and the resultant recruitment difficulties have meant that many front-line child protection workers have insufficient knowledge, skills, and training to undertake this complex work. Denying inexperienced staff access to information that will assist them to make more reliable decisions seems counterproductive. However, in our view, the central issue surrounding use of risk assessment instruments, or the English Assessment of Need instrument for that matter, is the propensity for them to be used routinely and uncritically by professional staff as a means to routinize decision making and working relationships with children and parents (Cooper *et al.* 2003).

Sophisticated ICT systems are incorporated into case management practices and, besides their client-related functions, are usually employed to increase staff compliance with the organization's key policies and procedures, for example, how frequently case planning is undertaken, and the standardization of assessments of risk, need, and service eligibility. ICT's have had profound effects on the roles and duties of professional staff, increasing the auditing and surveillance functions through the sharing and monitoring of information about groups deemed to be dangerous (Parton 2007). While, arguably, case management systems have promoted consistency of service delivery, there has also been criticism that this has led to undue proceduralism and a subsequent lack of creativity by professional staff (Froggett 2002; Cooper *et al.* 2003). Some writers have also argued that case management systems have become too management-driven as opposed to professionally directed and that risk management strategies have become pervasive and counterproductive to proactive professional resourcefulness in problem solving (Howe 1994; Froggett 2002; Lonne and Thomson 2005). In essence, a routinized "off the shelf" approach is taken too far in too many cases, with creative and beneficial work with children and families occurring because of the skills and inclinations of committed staff rather than the program and policy principles and approaches. Too often help is provided to those in dire need despite the system, rather than because of it. Taken overall, while case management has been beneficial to performance measurement and management, it has been retrograde in the critical element of worker–client relations, the key to facilitating the changes necessary to address and prevent child abuse and neglect (Cooper *et al.* 2003).

When examined overall, it is apparent that NPM has had a critical influence on child protection systems through key elements such as setting clear program outcomes and targets, the central role of case management, the use of a range of audit and surveillance processes, utilization of sophisticated client and management information systems, and the assessment of risk and need, often through a creeping proceduralism that has accompanied detailed policy directives. For example, the Assessment Framework in England and tools such as Structured Decision Making in the USA and Australia have been promoted by NPM advocates as necessary for quality practice even though the programs in these countries have quite different foci and emphases in attending to prevention of abuse and neglect. NPM has had a pervasive influence partly because it has been flexibly adapted to different community, organizational, and program contexts. It has been a key factor in the creeping proceduralization of child protection work, often at the expense of more relationship-based practice.

Working in child protection

Working in child protection is a vocation for many, if not most, practitioners—a labor of love that entails immense compassion, caring and commitment to children and their parents and families (Anderson 2000; McLean and Andrew 2000; Mor Barak *et al.* 2001; Savicki 2002; Weaver *et al.* 2007). However, there are indications that social workers have experienced a more difficult occupation following the rise of neoliberal managerialist agendas, with increased stress from above, rampant bureaucracy and paperwork, and service delivery adversely affected by agency practices, procedures, and budgets (Aronson and Sammon 2000; Jones 2001; Gupta and Blewett 2007). For many child protection practitioners, practice is made deeply distressing by their exposure to the power-laden, abusive and unhealthy organizational environments that they work in (Aronson and Sammon 2000; Jones 2001). It is little wonder that for many staff, their stint in child protection is cut short because of the inherent difficulties associated with: dealing with people who are in extreme need, have multiple social and personal problems, and who are often prone to anger; excessively high work demands; a general lack of support and understanding from management; and organizational cultures and climates that are hostile and conflictual (Jones 2001; Savicki 2002; Stanley and Goddard 2002; Bednar 2003; Smith and Donovan 2003; Smith 2005; Gupta and Blewett 2007; Weaver *et al.* 2007). A common explanation for staff departure is that these individuals failed to cope with the difficult nature of the work. We suggest that they are better viewed as casualties of an unhealthy system, in a way that strangely parallels that of the children and families exposed to it.

Many people, of course, have lengthy and satisfying careers in child protection and develop high level skills and knowledge that are the cornerstone of the many successes that are achieved. Unfortunately, when examined globally, job dissatisfaction in child protection systems is too high and the related high staff turnover is endemic and unsustainable, although exceptions are notable in some European countries (Savicki 2002; Hill *et al.* 2002). This is not just the result of failures in HRM systems and the associated discourse, but of a total organizational environment that is failing and, in some instances, is abusive toward its employees. We now turn the spotlight on the research about the organizational environments of child protection practice.

Understanding the nature of the work roles and tasks is critical to any analysis of the organizational environment of child protection systems. Essentially, child protection practitioners receive uncertain, complex and incomplete information about the circumstances of children and families; they apply professional knowledge to ascertain if they are at "risk" or "in need"; contact those involved and utilize high level interpersonal skills in order to learn about their intimate and complex lives and relationships; assess the information in light of relevant laws, policy, and procedures; then make decisions which may have profound impacts on their lives and for which they are accountable to others; and then implement these (hopefully) wise decisions in order to enhance the safety and well-being of those who are vulnerable to abuse and neglect (Turnell and Edwards 1999). All this occurs within a dynamic set of relationships at the macro, mezzo and micro levels, with diversity of gender, cultures, ages, and personalities apparent. Personal values and beliefs, and raw emotions, are critical elements. Conflicts abound in what is a fluid and uncertain set of events. Questions as to which is the best course of action are riven with the possibility, usually low, of dire outcomes for those who are involved. Saying it is difficult work is a serious understatement. It is apparent that to do this sort of work people must be committed, talented and well-trained, personally resilient to work-related stress, and well supported (Anderson 2000; Weaver *et al.* 2007).

There is considerable importance in the vocational motivations of those who choose this work, with a number of studies highlighting the critical importance of personal commitment to the job as an aid to job satisfaction and a buffer for work stress and associated staff turnover (Anderson 2000; McLean and Andrew 2000; Dollard *et al.* 2001; Mor Barak *et al.* 2001; Lonne 2003; Weaver *et al.* 2007). While recognizing that it is a tough occupation, people generally choose this line of work because they feel they can make a positive difference in the lives of others, particularly those who are vulnerable and disadvantaged. Altruism is an important element of their motivation, whereas financial remuneration is typically of much lesser importance (Lonne 2003). They are ideal sorts of employees as their commitment means that they are frequently prepared to put up with difficulties and disappointments and "go the extra mile." However, despite these high levels of vocational commitment, many soon find that the job is simply not worth it and leave. Documented rates of turnover are unsustainably high (Jones 2001; Anderson and Gobeil 2002; Savicki 2002; Bednar 2003; Gupta and Blewett 2007; Testro and Peltola 2007; Weaver *et al.* 2007).

So why do they depart in such numbers? The reasons are complex and interrelated but the research evidence is clear that it is primarily the result of organizational factors rather than individual or community ones (Dollard *et al.* 2001; Mor Barak *et al.* 2001; Savicki 2002; Bednar 2003; Lonne 2003; Ellett *et al.* 2007). Job satisfaction is inversely related with work stress, which has a strong positive relationship with staff turnover (Mor Barak *et al.* 2001; Bednar 2003; Weaver *et al.* 2007). The typical process is for high demand organizational and work factors to occur; staff are given insufficient support and work stress rises along with job dissatisfaction; a trigger incident occurs and workers decide to leave (Dollard *et al.* 2001). Taken overall, the following factors are critical influences on work stress:

- role ambiguity, confusion and conflict associated with an unclear social mandate, high expectations and unclear responsibilities, and insufficient direction from the organization regarding competing priorities (Savicki 2002; Lonne 2003; Gupta and Blewett 2007; Weaver *et al.* 2007);

- high and unsustainable workloads are experienced due to under-resourcing, existing staff shortages and the continued rise in child protection reports that require investigation and statutory intervention (Anderson and Gobeil 2002; D. Scott 2006a);
- lack of autonomy in the work role associated with increased procedural-ization and routinization of work tasks, along with decreased professional discretion (Dollard *et al.* 2001; Lonne 2003; Gupta and Blewett 2007);
- management that is overly outcome-focused and driven by high expecta-tions of efficiency and performance, and yet is unsupportive of stressed staff (Mor Barak *et al.* 2001; Lonne 2003; Gupta and Blewett 2007);
- strained organizational cultures and climates that are characterized by high levels of structural and interpersonal tension, conflict, and change, with resultant distrust affecting communication (Cooper *et al.* 2003);
- conflictual staff–service user relations, including threats, violence and ex-posure to client tragedies, hurt and critical incidents (Stanley and Goddard 2002; Regehr *et al.* 2004; Smith *et al.* 2004; Littlechild 2005; Dumbrill 2006); and
- lack of perceived work success as unsuccessful interventions tend to lead to service users remaining in contact, while those who have had effective interventions disappear from view (Lonne 2003).

In fact, there is compelling evidence that the level of staff turnover is so high as to make staffing the key organizational issue in child protection systems, which depend upon highly skilled and experienced staff to under-take successful interventions (Shireman 2003). For example, Bednar (2003) cites rates between 46 and 90 percent of staff leaving within a two-year period in the USA. There are similar problems elsewhere (Anderson and Gobeil 2002; Cooper *et al.* 2003; Morris 2005; Smith 2005; Glisson *et al.* 2006; Nunno 2006; Ellett *et al.* 2007; Gupta and Blewett 2007; Weaver *et al.* 2007), particularly in rural and remote locations (Lonne and Cheers 2004a,b; Cheers *et al.* 2007).

Unfortunately, the high staff turnover produces a circular problem: workers leave due to high workload and dissatisfaction; vacancies then exist which increases the workload pressures on remaining staff; workers continue to leave due to high workload; other professionals and the community hears about the workload problems and high turnover, which leads to decreased interest in the work and problematic recruitment; staff shortages continue and lead to chronic workload problems. Moreover, having a continual influx of inexperi-enced and often recently trained staff to fill vacancies has a detrimental impact on the knowledge and skills level of the agency, and can compound the prob-lems by detracting from the agency's reputation. Agencies have, of course, devoted huge resources and effort to address these problems, with mixed suc-cess but no overall solutions. The situation persists despite these valiant attempts at finding and successfully implementing remedial strategies.

The push toward child protection specialization and resultant human resource issues has also had implications for the tertiary training of staff (Bellefeuille and Schmidt 2006), with calls for increased focus by educators upon developing skilled practitioners (Community Affairs Reference Committee, Australian Senate 2005; Healy and Meagher 2007; Gupta and Blewett 2007). There are identified problems in the quality of training programs both internal and external to agencies (Nunno 2006; Healy and Meagher 2007), which may contribute to a perception of falling practice standards. Despite the fact that many good-hearted and talented people are committed to preventing children from being abused and neglected, the recruitment and retention, and training problems being experienced are making it less possible to provide a system that can achieve this (Shireman 2003).

The recruitment difficulties are being addressed in some locations by extending the acceptable qualifications from the traditional social work and welfare professionals to a much broader human service pool and even wider. While understandable, this strategy seems short-sighted and only likely to exacerbate the existing problems. Some researchers have argued that there is an already increasing trend in the human services toward de-professionalization (Healy and Meagher 2004; Meagher and Healy 2006). There is a wealth of research evidence which demonstrates the need for greater attention upon staff relational skills and knowledge base about the factors associated with child abuse and neglect and how to effectively assist people to change (Froggett 2002; Cooper *et al.* 2003; Blewett *et al.* 2007; Gupta and Blewett 2007). Effective interventions require much more than a good heart and a commitment to children's welfare. It is exceptionally complex work that requires talented practitioners who have high level interpersonal skills and the requisite knowledge and support (Turnell and Edwards 1999; Healy and Meagher 2007). Staffing a child protection system with people who are out of their depth and blindly follow procedures is a recipe for disaster, with serious consequences for children and families.

Although many child protection workers hold qualifications other than social work, in some jurisdictions the values and wholistic practice framework of this profession has been instrumental in promoting social justice for those who are most likely to come into contact with the child protection system— the poor, women, those with disabilities, and other disadvantaged groups, including Indigenous peoples and people of color (Shireman 2003; Healy and Meagher 2007). As we will argue in the second part of this book, for all its shortcomings as a profession, the underpinning values and ethical framework of social work has an important part to play in realigning child protection systems into a more humane social institution that provides children and families with constructive interventions into their lives. Moreover, social work practice principles have much to offer the dysfunctional cultures and climates that currently pervade these chronically failing organizations (Lonne and Thomson 2005).

Organizational cultures and climates

We have suggested that, generally speaking, child protection systems are failing yet continue to persist in their endeavors. We have also examined the changed role and functions of social welfare systems and the impact of NPM on these and on child protection systems. The research on work stress, job satisfaction and turnover demonstrates that many staff experience a very difficult work environment, often resulting in departure. But what parts do organizational culture and climate play in this dynamic equation? Glisson and Hemmelgarn contend:

> Caseworkers must perform their jobs in highly stressful situations that can involve, for example, angry family members or seriously emotionally disturbed children. Therefore, the levels of conflict, role clarity, job satis- faction, cooperation, personalization, and other variables that charac- terize the shared attitudes and climate of their work environments should be powerful determinants of how caseworkers respond to unexpected problems, the tenacity with which difficult problems are solved, and the affective tone of their work-related interactions with children and families.
>
> (Glisson and Hemmelgarn 1998: 404)

In a rigorous follow-up study, Glisson *et al.* (2006) found caseworker turnover was reduced by two-thirds following a year-long involvement into urban and rural children's services case management teams in the USA by experienced staff trained in the use of the availability, responsiveness and continuity (ARC) organizational intervention. The ARC depends on general systems theory and focuses on providing clear guidance and support to staff through promotion of guiding principles including being mission-driven, results-oriented, improvement-directed, relationship-centered, and participation-based. It is a multi-tiered holistic intervention that utilizes collaborative participation and promotes innovations in work and management practices. The study demonstrated that organizational climate was significantly im- proved by reducing role conflict, role overload, emotional exhaustion, and depersonalization.

Organizational climate can be defined as the attitudes shared by employees about their current environment (Glisson and Hemmelgarn 1998: 404). It is a key influence upon organizational culture and vice versa. Organizational climate will tend to ebb and flow depending on the events taking place and how these are perceived and affect employees and key external groups (social actors), such as children and families in child protection systems. For example, when the media is attacking a child protection agency about a child death or scandal, the climate may be very defensive and resistant to suggestions of poor practice. Climate may be somewhat transitory depending on current events, but it is strongly influenced by the underlying organizational culture, and it is an important determinant of the organization's effectiveness, particularly service quality and outcomes for children and families (Glisson and Hemmelgarn 1998; Glisson *et al.* 2006).

On the other hand, organizational culture is comprised of the sum total of the values, beliefs and ideologies of the people who make it up and has been defined as "the patterned ways that an organization responds to its challenges, whether these are explicit (for example a crisis) or implicit (a latent problem or opportunity)" (Westrum 2004: 22). It has a number of sources including national culture, sector values, professional values and individual beliefs (Thompson *et al.* 1996). For example, a strong cultural belief in many child protection agencies is that they are the "good guys," who embrace noble values such as helping the vulnerable and bringing aid to the suffering.

However, there is no single organizational culture within a specific agency, although there may be dominant ones, subservient ones, emerging, and subversive ones. There is a variety of cultures and sub-cultures that operate, each with its own narratives (stories) and ways of perceiving and interpreting their world. For example, in an early study of three social services departments in the UK, Kakabadse (1982) found that front-line staff culture tended to be primarily motivated by practice- and client-related values, whereas middle management were frequently more concerned with organizational role and functional matters, and senior management embraced a power culture that included an external and politically sensitive orientation. For an organization to be effective and successful, its cultures must be congruent in relation to their core values and beliefs about the agency mission and objectives. Meyer and Zucker (1989) noted that when there is significant conflict between various cultural groupings, organizations will struggle to be efficient and perform effectively.

Apart from the climate, organizational cultures in statutory child protection agencies and systems are influenced by a range of key factors including:

- the cultural make up and values within the society, including dominant attitudes toward social care and the social construction of children and families (Mildred 2003; Ferguson 2004; Holland and Scourfield 2004; France and Utting 2005; Merrick 2006; Parton 2006a);
- the legal framework and specific authority that empowers the agency to intervene (Cheers *et al.* 2007);
- the agency's mission and objectives and the extent to which these are shared by the various groups and social actors within and external to it (Meyer and Zucker 1989; Jones and May 1992; Westrum 2004);
- the leadership of the agency and its attitudes to staff and other social actors (Anheier 1999; Jones 2001; Cooper *et al.* 2003; Crime and Misconduct Commission (CMC) 2004; Barton and Welbourne 2005);
- the dominant discourses adopted by professionals as to the best ways to protect children, promote child and family well-being, and their approaches to the use of power and authority that shape staff–client relationships (Chevannes 2002; Dawson and Berry 2002; Smith and

Donovan 2003; Holland and Scourfield 2004; Morris 2005; Glisson *et al.* 2006); and

- day-to-day workload and practice crises, in particular placement break-downs, that end with distressed and angry parents, children and carers offloading emotionally to harried workers, resulting in further stress (Wilson *et al.* 2000; Gilbertson and Barber 2003, 2004; Regehr *et al.* 2004; Smith *et al.* 2004; Spratt and Callan 2004; Littlechild 2005).

We contend that across most Western nations, but not all, the contemporary dominance of neoconservative social attitudes and neoliberal values that steer social welfare (workfare), has led to a blaming, punitive and socially divisive ideology prevailing, leaving little room for notions of social care as opposed to social control (Parton 1996; Chevannes 2002; Dawson and Berry 2002; Smith and Donovan 2003; McDonald 2006; Pelton 2008). The social mission for social welfare and, in particular, child protection has come to act as a surveillance system upon those sections of the community who are perceived as dangerous, troublesome or dependent—groups such as the poor, single-parents who are mostly women, people of color, and other minority racial groupings, Indigenous people, and those with disabilities (Shireman 2003). Unfortunately, child protection systems tend to investigate and assess rather than provide assistance to those in need (Melton and Thompson 2002; Shireman 2003; Melton 2005), a system that has been promoted under the guise of a child safety (saving) rhetoric (Merrick 2006).

The primary cultural behavior is the legally sanctioned use of authority and the overuse (abuse) of power. There are a series of parallel processes with this use of power. The politicization of public sectors has witnessed politicians and their minders clearly exercising political power over child protection agencies, quite often using the language of "accountability" and "reform" (Walter 2006). Senior executives then wield power over middle managers to meet performance measures that bear little resemblance to the actualities of the work, yet domination of these lower-level supervisors often occurs with the velvet glove, and an implicit threat of adverse consequences for "poor performance" (Tilbury 2006; Wells 2006). These harried and stressed supervisors are then apt to parallel this abuse of power with their front-line staff, showing this by often not providing the support they need, being directive and demanding in their relations, and unsympathetic when paper-work is not completed on time or targets are not met. It is unsurprising that the abuse of power and punitive attitudes are then often paralleled when child protection workers undertake intrusive investigations ever mindful of the need to quickly get the facts and move on to the next report and assess-ment, but also uneasy about the lack of space and time given to relationship building with the parents and children they are supposed to be helping (Turnell and Edwards 1999). All this is compounded by care placement breakdowns and emergencies, which in many ways drives a culture and climate of perma-nent crisis. Organizational culture in child protection systems has a direct and profound bearing on the outcomes for children and families (Glisson and Hemmelgarn 1998; Glisson *et al.* 2006).

These parallel processes of abusive power and crisis may typify the relations within child protection systems, but it needs to be made clear that many staff at all levels find these approaches repugnant, and refuse to act this way and try valiantly to resist them. That specific interventions, teams, work units, programs, and agencies are able to work differently and provide high level care and effective helping, and facilitate significant positive change in the lives of people, families, neighborhoods, and communities is testament to their compassion, commitment, and competence. They demonstrate that there are alternative and better ways.

Another key aspect of dysfunctional child protection systems stems from the incongruent discourses often held by senior management, middle management, and front-line staff (CMC 2004). We have already outlined NPM and its dominant values and practices. In our view, the language used in child protection systems to describe and implement managerial direction, control, and monitoring (e.g. performance measurement, risk assessment) does not resonate well with most professional staff. Instead, practitioners tend to use the language and conceptual frameworks of their professional training (e.g. cognitive behavioral, systems theory and family therapy, strengths-based) and remain client-oriented (usually child-centered but not always family-focused) (Froggett 2002). Middle managers are critical mediators and interpreters of both downward and upward communications, without which there would likely be a fundamental breakdown in relations. This has on occasions occurred of course, leading to public inquiries or staff industrial action.

While there is significant diversity, taken overall, the climate within child protection systems, we contend, reflects the blaming and punitive conservative values and distrust of professionals that we have outlined earlier. There is a negative effect on staff from media frenzies that seek to highlight systemic failings and discrete cases where the outcomes are harmful for those concerned, especially children (Hill 1990; Holland and Scourfield 2004; Rustin 2004; Butler and Drakeford 2005; Connolly and Doolan 2006, 2007). Defensiveness abounds and tends to shut down reflection and dialogue about the vexed issues at hand. Examined systemically, the defensiveness can show itself as a "closed system," reinforced when politicians react to critical incidents with ever more strident language about protecting every child from risk, an unrealistic expectation and literal impossibility. Meanwhile executives, managers, and practitioners feel fatigued from continual organizational restructurings and policy change, and resign themselves to continued scapegoating from an anxious public and media.

It is ironic that many inquiries into systemic failings and child deaths have, among other things, identified the need for cultural change in child protection agencies but have not been as able to articulate the incongruencies between the various articulations of what the mission of child protection agencies should be. In our view, child protection systems have demonstrated themselves to be chronically failing, despite numerous wholehearted attempts at reform to make them work effectively. Their missions are too broad and ambiguous, with numerous social actors having input, and their continued low performance persisting. Their cultures and climates are often destructive to those who work in them or come into contact with them. In the second part of the book we will put forward a new approach that addresses the issues raised.

5 Service users and stakeholders

In this chapter we examine the collective experiences of, and issues for, service users and a variety of other stakeholders in contemporary Anglophone child protection systems. In some senses, the groups we include here sit uneasily in a chapter together. Service users, professionals, community groups, and other stakeholders are powerfully aware of the different spaces they occupy in the context of twenty-first century child protection systems. Each of these stakeholders may be committed to competing positions on vitally important subjects including ones such as what constitutes adequate care, parent and child rights, the meaning of "the best interests of the child," family responsibilities and family autonomy, and the role of the state. They may well share some common goals but may believe in very different means for achieving them. The very nature of child protection is that most stakeholders involved in such systems and activities experience considerable pain and distress, stemming from different experiences of, and perspectives on, the complex and difficult events that occur, and from the challenging stressors in the myriad relationships they have to manage. Child protection systems always deal with vulnerable people (children and adults) in highly emotional states in extremely contested human environments.

The rationale behind including service users', practitioners' and others' perspectives in the same chapter is that they are significant stakeholders in a system that often has major adverse impacts on all groups. The inclusion of their experiences and perspectives in the one chapter helps to elucidate the competing forces in child welfare practice and will contribute significantly to a well-articulated vision for an alternative system. It is not argued here that their experiences can be conflated and homogenized. For example, professionals cannot speak adequately for parents (Testro and Peltola 2007). They cannot speak adequately for children either. Valuable insights can emerge from hearing the oft competing voices of those involved.

Many writers view the term "service user" and "parent" synonymously. We argue that the voices of a variety of groups, beginning with children and young people themselves, should be seen as service users in child protection. While the term "service user" has commonly been applied to parents, we believe that an understanding of notions of service users in child protection must start with children and young people. Although children and young people are the focus, there is essentially an adult-centric orientation in child protection (Irwin *et al.* 2006), with adults frequently speaking "for" children and young people, who are often the passive recipients of considerable activity around their needs.

In light of their frequent sidelining, we begin with children and young people, and span out to those adults around them whose voices should also be heard. These groups are parents and extended family members, foster carers, child protection practitioners, and a range of other community stakeholders. Nevertheless, it is important to also avoid blurring the boundaries around the situations of other stakeholders in child protection systems. Perspectives can be very different but insight into each of them is valuable in conceptualizing child protection reform. For example, Dumbrill's (2006) study of parents' narratives found that they valued recognition by workers of the power relations inherent in child protection proceedings. Postmodern perspectives on power are very useful in this area, as adopting binary oppositionality of stakeholders in child protection is unhelpful and inaccurate (Healy 1998).

To fully operationalize a commitment to a service user oriented approach in child protection work would necessitate restructuring the child protection system to include broader structural and social changes. Such reforms would probably entail a rebalancing of the social and other relations inherent within current Anglophone market-dominated polities, which are characterized by high levels of privatization, a severe cleavage in the life circumstances of the well-off and the poor, and a tendency toward highly residualized systems of welfare provision. This is the broader environment in which these child protection services are located (Maluccio *et al.* 2000). For example, Cooper notes that:

> The key principles upon which an effective and responsive child protec-
> tion system must rest concern issues of trust, authority and negotiation.
> These concepts seem to us to encapsulate features which have been
> weakened and eroded in recent decades in England and Wales, and perhaps
> other parts of the UK yet are strengths of other European countries.
>
> (A. Cooper 2002: 131)

Limitations of the literature

Most research studies into disparate human experiences are small scale and this is the case in the child protection field broadly, and specifically in the material presented around service users and practitioners. Hence, caution should be exercised in extrapolating the findings presented in this chapter into generalizations. Rather, the findings should be viewed as important illustrations of the diverse experiences of those caught up in these systems.

Relationship

Relationship is a lens to view the narratives and stories that follow. Relationships are essential for effective helping; yet, relationships that are necessary for effective helping are frequently not possible in the current system or are, at least, quite difficult and highly dependent on the approach of individuals. We agree with Ruch, who asserts that "In order for relationship-based practice to develop and flourish, the uncertainty and anxiety associated with the emotionally charged subject matter that social work comprises must be effectively addressed" (Ruch 2005: 111). Understanding human behavior only at a rational level discounts the value of narrative, because narrative stems from the meaning people give to their lived experiences. This is no less true in child protection than in any other context, including those in which human services work occurs.

Cultural issues

Cultural difference is an area where child protection policy and practice has, at the very least, faltered and frequently failed children and families. For example, the resounding call from Indigenous peoples is for child protection authorities to fully appreciate that Western approaches to child protection based on an individualist and atomistic approach to "the child" have little or no synergy with Indigenous values of family, community, and the connection with land. An Indigenous carer in an Australian study put it this way:

> You have to blame the parents for the abuse and neglect. A lot of people are not caring for the children. But when taking the children away, you can place them with an aunty or relative. That relative might be the one to get the help for the mother. The help should be there for the parents as well as the children. They just look at taking the children away but don't think about what's left. Later on that child will go back to that root. So we need to not let that root die.
>
> (Higgins *et al.* 2006: 45)

The seriousness of the plight of Indigenous children should not be underestimated because the patterns of Indigenous dispossession are similar in North America, Australia and New Zealand, with profound consequences for these peoples. Hart (2002) and Proulx and Perrault (2000) emphasize a full engagement with families and communities, but an unwavering commitment to the protection of children. In a Canadian study, one young person said:

> It was very lonely . . . a lot of neglect and sexual abuse—and physical— no stability, very dysfunctional family.
>
> (Proulx and Perrault 2000: 45)

Another remarked:

> My older sister knew and all she did—I was made to feel so bad—I told
> the priest I had sex (but I had been raped). It was really sad. I didn't realize
> back then that I was a victim. I don't know, making a child feel so bad.
>
> (Proulx and Perrault 2000: 45)

Aboriginal approaches emphasize the spiritual needs of families and communities, and advocate the use of spiritual knowledge in bringing about
positive change. It is crucial to listen to the stories behind the family problems
resulting in child abuse and neglect, and to locate these in the disconnection
from culture that is almost always present (Churchill 1994; Hart 2002). One
of the difficulties for Indigenous people is that many workers in Western
jurisdictions can understand the importance of cultural awareness in a
workshop setting, but have trouble in applying this knowledge when relating
with families. Unfortunately, past mistakes have currency in the present child
protection jurisdictions located in Anglophone countries. Developing an
understanding of how these factors play out for children and families is a key
theme in this book. We argue for a more family-inclusive approach regardless
of the cultural background of children and young people. However, the effects
of culturally alien concepts of family and community in the lives of Indigenous
children are particularly problematic.

Children and young people

When we write of service users we must begin with children and young people
in the child protection system. In many other contexts of their lives, the issues
of parents and other family members themselves are central. However, when
we are considering child protection, the focus must be the children and young
people for whom these systems exist, and the care work is done. Locating children centrally is a moral imperative due to their vulnerability and general lack
of power in Anglophone societies. The discourses of children and young people
have shaped contemporary child protection practice and illustrate the power
of narrative in informing knowledge to improve practice and policy. These
discourses typically depict dominant narratives about family, the passivity of
children and young people as victims, and the ways in which interventions
to ensure protection take place in their lives. An alternative and inclusive
approach is growing in influence in research-informed practice and policy
(Mason and Gibson 2004).

An English study by Leeson (2007) sought the narratives of young people
in care in order to consider what workers need to bear in mind to hear
children's voices, understand the ethical issues in dealing with children and
young people in care and their distress, and engage with them in their care.
Leeson found that workers frequently made most decisions for children in
relation to their participation in her study and generally around issues to do
with their lives. Four key themes emerged:

1   A sense of helplessness experienced by children who were not involved in decisions about their own lives but, rather, had decisions made for them;

2   A conviction by children and young people that 'corporate parenting' did not meet their needs;

3   A valuing of workers if they acted consistently, were concerned for children, and acted as advocates; and

4   An expressed view that attempts to communicate how they were feeling had met with a lack of understanding from the adults concerned. Young people were frequently labeled as badly behaved rather than having their reactions understood as an expression of distress and a sense of powerlessness.

(Leeson 2007)

In order to expand on these ideas we have discussed children's narratives in terms of the subjective meaning they give to their own experiences. Parton (2006a) found that children and young people felt that their own wishes around what should be done about disclosures were frequently discounted and that adults either trivialized or exaggerated events, taking decisions for children and young people about actions to be taken that were at odds with their preferences.

It is important to also capture the experiences of children not in statutory systems but deemed at risk and therefore in contact with these systems. The experiences of these children and young people are also frequently quite negative. Irwin *et al.* (2006) argued for the involvement of children and young people in research on domestic violence, and highlighted the following young person's statement.

Some kids will open up if they trust someone. But if no one's talking to them and no one's saying that they're here for you, they're not going to say anything. No one told me that they would listen.

(Irwin *et al.* 2006: 22)

When adults listen to the experiences of children and young people who are caught up in the statutory child protection system, they learn that children and young people find the systems adult-centric (Irwin *et al.* 2006). There is a disturbing lack of faith held by many children in the ability of those in formal systems to help them in serious situations. For example, Wattam's (2002) research found that children themselves make less than 5 percent of referrals to statutory services. The overwhelming majority of referrals come from adults, and then, it is concerned professionals in the greatest numbers, with fewer referrals coming from family members and others.

Mudaly and Goddard (2006) explored children's views of the abuse they experienced and their experience of professional interventions and suggested that professionals can contribute to the silencing of children's voices.

> I mean people like that are supposed to listen, they're not supposed to sit there and tell you what you're thinking or what you're feeling, because that's what she was doing just sitting there and telling me what's right.

And furthermore:

> As far as I am concerned, and sorry for saying this, but if you ask me ... you know that the system is well and truly stuffed.
>
> (Mudaly and Goddard 2006: 104)

Generally speaking, young people leaving state care and protection systems in Anglophone countries have significantly poorer life outcomes as measured across a range of economic, social and health indicators (Stein 2006). Compared to their peers who are not in care, they experience higher unemployment and lower incomes, poorer educational achievements, and have higher levels of mental illness, including depression and substance abuse, bear their own children while at a younger age, and have increased contact with the criminal justice system (Pecora *et al.* 2003, 2005, 2006; Courtney and Dworsky 2006; Stein 2006; Wade and Dixon 2006; Berridge 2007). They are significantly more likely to experience homelessness and its consequences, particularly if they have had high levels of placement instability and breakdown while in care (Gilbertson and Barber 2003; Mendes and Moslehuddin 2004; Mendes 2005; Wade and Dixon 2006). This happens despite a raft of changes and reforms to alternative care systems, including increased access to required resources and help, and enhanced systems of accountability (Shireman 2003; Gilbertson and Barber 2004). Sadly, many young people are discharged from care into insecure accommodation and can experience bouts of homelessness in their transition from care, particularly when there has been a failure to adequately assess their capability to live independently and access suitable supports and housing arrangements (Mendes and Moslehuddin 2004; Courtney and Dworsky 2006). Conversely, those young people who have the opportunity to remain living with their foster family fare better in the transition to independence (Courtney and Dworsky 2006).

Care systems differ across jurisdictions, and alternatives to those found in Anglophone countries are found in some Western European countries. These are generally characterized by an advanced commitment to the rights and needs of children and young people that is located in an institutional framework, which values respect for children and invests heavily in state programs. The very existence of a range of alternatives, beginning with intensive in-home responses and including innovative residential options along with foster care, is an indication of a sophisticated way of thinking about the needs of children and young people (Hessle 2000; Hill *et al.* 2002). An example countering the adult-centric nature of conventional approaches is Kinderhaus, a residential facility in Germany where active choice by children and young people is a hallmark characteristic. Such approaches sit within a collaboratively oriented and voluntary system.

> If a placement in care is decided by a court or by a specially-assigned guardian, the family has the legal right to express their wishes or their choice . . . If the children are old enough, they can assess the options and choose the one they are happiest with. The child or young person does not have to make their decision in front of their parents.
>
> (International Movement ATD Fourth World 2004: 139)

A report by the Children's Rights Director for England (Morgan 2007) used web surveys and discussion groups seeking the views of children and young people regarding what kept them safe. A number of issues were canvassed and, again, the message was delivered unambiguously that children and young people want to be listened to. One wrote to the web survey that in order to be heard, "we should be aloud" (sic) (Morgan 2007: 18). Another said that "if people come to you with choices they should also help you make sense of them" (Morgan 2007: 18).

The message that children and young people want to be heard, and are frequently misunderstood by workers and judged harshly (Leeson 2007) has been heeded in an Australian paper entitled *Every Child Every Chance* (2007), which calls for a much higher level of understanding than currently exists in relation to the way trauma and abuse are manifested in children's reactions. In keeping with an emphasis on relationship:

> Outcomes for children will be enhanced if we take the time and remain open to hearing the voice and experience of the child . . . Interventions need to be both engaging of families and forensically astute . . . practitioners need to listen to the voice of the child and seek to understand the language of their behaviour.
>
> (Victorian Government Department of Human Services 2007: 44)

The theme of engaging with children is critically important and there is much more to be done if we are to appreciate the importance of framing child protection systems in Anglophone societies within this approach.

Parents

It is clear that there are many positive stories about parental experiences with child protection systems and that staff are, by and large, dedicated and committed to trying to make things better for parents and children. For example, in Dale's (2004) study on family experiences one parent said: "We've been very lucky—he's great. He's been very helpful, his mannerism

—we've even looked forward to him coming. He's not treated us like criminals—not like how we felt treated at first" (Dale 2004: 150).

Nevertheless, within proceduralized and bureaucratized systems that investigate rather than provide help, many parents find the contact with child protection workers to be a negative experience. We contend that the predominant systemic discourses and approaches have a significant influence on shaping the social relations between practitioners and parents, with the end result too often being counterproductive to effectively protecting children. Engaging successfully with parents requires skilled staff—the lynch pin to good practice. Unfortunately, in contemporary child protection systems, too often people are helped despite the system rather than because of it.

Within the framework of these relationships, we favor the concept of "partnership" with service users, particularly parents, over that of participation. Participation can connote a partial or conditional involvement, devised and managed by a dominant party. In the context of child protection, it is more useful to put forward the concept of partnership between service users and practitioners as it appears to have more potential to be anti-oppressive (Dumbrill 2003). Nevertheless, it is important to avoid the pitfalls inherent in a romanticized view about partnership with parents whose children are the subject of statutory child protection involvement. Healy (1998) alerts us to the difficulties of migrating generic concepts of partnership, theorized in positive terms, from other contexts where the stakes may not be as critically high as they are when protecting children.

People do not usually elect to have lifelong careers as service users. However, many do experience lengthy disadvantage, which is sometimes transgenerational. For many parents, life continues to be a great struggle before, during and after the intervention of statutory child protection services. In addition, as a result of the way child protection is framed in the current risk-averse climate, there is often little incentive or encouragement for workers to pursue partnerships with parents of children in care. Indeed, because of the nature of the system where aversion of risk is uppermost (Scourfield and Welsh 2003), when workers form strong relationships with parents there are sometimes career penalties attached. They can be seen as "soft" on abuse (Dumbrill 2003), and there is little understanding of the potential to form strong helping relationships with parents, while at the same time, attending carefully and effectively to the needs of children (Trotter 2004; Thorpe 2007).

Testro and Peltola (2007) note that the assessment of risk to a child or children is often not compatible with assessing the needs of a family, particularly when the needs of vulnerable families far exceed the child protection system's capacity. This mismatch in needs and service responses is a fundamental problem in many child protection systems, and gives rise to much of the miscommunication that takes place between parents and those charged with operating the system and working with service users. Parents often speak of going to authorities for help with managing parenting and finding instead that they are subject to surveillance and control (Parton 2006a). Workers, too, can find themselves experiencing a sense of helplessness that they are not able to locate the kinds of services that the family needs to keep the child safe and to maximize the well-being of the family. Narrative portrayals are a powerful way to document the experiences of parents and Thorpe (2007) identified the following key themes:

- power
- lack of respect
- blame
- cultural issues
- lack of help, and
- the impact of disenfranchised grief.

Power

In many accounts, parents express anger and resentment about the ways in which workers in child protection settings "use" power, with many parents experiencing it as the antithesis of partnership.

> One parent spoke of needing to know the rules of the power game: I would have been humbled a long time ago . . . I would have kissed their arses, bowed, whatever.
>
> (McCullum 1995 cited in Dumbrill 2003: 109)

> The worst thing? The threats, behaviour, power they've got. The big words they used frightened me—really frightened me . . . arrogant, veryarrogant. Ignorant as well. That person's approach: She didn't ask, she told.
>
> (Dale 2004: 50)

Lack of respect

Parents have spoken of frequently feeling that they are not seen as worthy of respect and fair treatment because they have been the caregivers of children who have required care from the state. Parents have cited calls not being returned, visits with children being cancelled without explanation and not rescheduled, and documentation of formal processes not being provided. Parents have spoken of meetings about their children (which should include them) proceeding in their absence when workers have made only cursory efforts to facilitate their involvement. Adverse judgments can be made about lack of commitment to their children when parents need flexibility around meetings to fit in with work or other appointments.

Blame

Within risk-averse and adversarial systems, parents often feel blamed and as though there is little understanding of the circumstances that have led to their children and their families becoming involved with authorities.

> I have this parental guilt and (child welfare) are great at piling it on higher. I live with the harshest judge of all, which is myself. I had a worker once who told me, "We know this (having son placed in a foster home) is an easy way out for you. You just do not want to parent your child." I had enough guilt over my inability to parent my child without someone telling me this.
>
> (de Boer and Coady 2007: 36)

Cultural issues

The importance of cultural issues has specific relevance for understanding the perspectives of parents. Thorpe (2007) identifies that parents from Indigenous or culturally and linguistically diverse (CALD) communities frequently feel judged by workers who lack cultural competence. Minimizing or dismissing outright the damaging effects of historical dispossession mixed with contemporary poverty often only results in judgment and blame.

Parents did not receive help

Not receiving required help is an enduring theme identified by many parents when they are asked about their perceptions and experiences of child protection interventions.

> I contacted social services for help, which did not come about for many, many months. I wanted advice—not getting any. Passed from pillar to post. They said they'd return calls—didn't return calls. Said they'd send people out—didn't. Social worker eventually turned up—I said "You're too late—I've been to hell and back."
>
> (Dale 2004: 144)

The way parents feel that they are approached and dealt with is also significant for them.

> If a social worker would have come to my door and rather than saying, "I'm here to check out a complaint," would say, "what do you need?" that would make all the difference. "I'm here because I want to help you keep things together."
>
> (Callahan and Lumb 1995: 804–5)

The impact of disenfranchised grief

Some parents experience "disenfranchised grief," defined as "a loss that is not or cannot be openly acknowledged, publicly mourned or socially supported" (Doka 1989: 4). The magnitude of losses to parents is often not appreciated by others. For parents, the loss of a child or children in these circumstances is painfully real. Yet, the grief and loss from having a child taken into state care because of problems in family care giving are not always seen as valid. A consistent theme in the experience of parents is this issue of unacknowledged grief, which is often minimized and misunderstood by workers operating from a deficit viewpoint about parents.

Other issues for parents

It is clear that many parents frequently feel differently than workers about the issues keeping their families in the child protection system. The terminology that workers use can be alienating to parents (Dale 2004), and is not always helpful in fostering productive relationships with them. For example, many parents dislike the formal language of classifications around "abuse," which for them carry meanings of deliberate and premeditated actions which were not their intention.

A Canadian study examining the situations of families seeking to stay together while involved with child protection authorities found that parents frequently feel that there is a resistance by workers to acknowledging their difficulties and their own needs which impact on their ability to care for their children.

> If my basic needs are met . . . I can care for my children . . . so many times I am tired, hungry . . . A lot of what we need is so basic . . . I need nurturing myself in order to parent.
>
> (Callahan and Lumb 1995: 804)

Parents who are "alumni" of the child protection system themselves (Pecora *et al.* 2003, 2005) often feel judged for this rather than it being acknowledged that their experiences have burdened them with extra difficulties that should be viewed with empathy rather than criticism. However, the use of risk assessment tools makes it very difficult for them to be judged on their current circumstances rather than just their past.

Gender and service user partnership

It is important to also acknowledge the gender dimension within service user experiences. A gap exists in the knowledge base in relation to the challenges to engaging fathers in most Anglophone countries and elsewhere (Pittman and Buckley 2006; Scourfield 2006). However, although somewhat problematically, fathers in England have had some success in being seen as stakeholders

(Featherstone 2004), while in many other locations there is little evidence of specific initiatives to work with fathers in ways that account for the gendered nature of family violence in the child protection context (Hickman 2003). Fathers are effectively "missing in action." We believe that fathers are important stakeholders in the protection of children and should be involved, along with mothers and other family members significant to children and young people. While mothers are frequently consulted by child protection authorities, albeit problematically, there is evidence to suggest that foster carers frequently have more say over decisions affecting children than their mothers, and certainly more than children's own social and biological fathers (Hansen and Ainsworth under review).

Featherstone (2004) has mounted a convincing argument that an avoidance of men as stakeholders in the child protection system places a huge burden on women as mothers because all the scrutiny falls on them, while men often escape the gaze. Writing about this issue some years ago in the UK context, and with the situation today still relatively unchanged in many other locations, Milner (1993) evocatively compares the child protection system which focuses only on mothers with:

> ... an elaborate and under funded ballet in which the mother pirouettes endlessly on worn out shoes without the support of a male partner. Indeed, whilst she attempts to undertake a pas de deux on her own, there is no criticism of the male lead who is off stage kicking the cygnets.
>
> (Milner 1993: 59)

Another important aspect of working with fathers is that often there also is no real engagement with them when they are not perpetrators of abuse against children. Responses to fathers can be one dimensional, epitomizing a rather binary classification of them as "bad" and mothers as "good," or at least "better than the father." However, while many fathers are able to be mobilized as protectors of children, their capacity to protect and nurture children is not optimized within this binary discourse.

Foster carers

Our framework does not include foster carers as service users. Rather, we contend that they should be acknowledged as part of the care team because their role is more akin to that of practitioners. Unfortunately, in many highly proceduralized systems of child protection carers do not fit easily in either group, their status being sometimes blurred and ambiguous. It is important to understand their situations because many systems have come to rely heavily on foster care for the care of children and young people apart from their families. Additionally, locating foster carers with practitioners can allow the focus to remain on children and young people within the context of their own families. It reinforces the earlier point about starting with children and young people and their networks, then moving to consideration of the narratives of workers and carers. We should not, however, ignore the fact that carers need access to resources in order to perform their roles and that they are sometimes seen as service users because they need to make material and other requests to assist in caring. A reformed system would make very clear the equitable partnership of foster carers and practitioners, despite this not always being an easy fit. This point does not, however, negate the importance of child protection workers engaging with the very difficult issues foster carers face, and using their skills as workers to assist them to address these.

There is considerable research into the experience of being a foster carer. For example Maclay *et al.* (2006) write about the quality of the relationship between foster carers and child protection workers. Carers reported frequently feeling unsupported and undervalued by statutory child protection practitioners. Fisher *et al.* (2000) studied carers' views of practitioners and found that support from them was deemed to be essential for carers to persevere with caring. In this UK study, carers valued three key areas in successful relationships with social workers. The first was physical and emotional availability: "He is very helpful. Supervises the contact and always keeps me informed" (Fisher *et al.* 2000: 227). The second and third areas in relation to worker input valued by foster carers were teamwork and respect; and help both of a practical nature and with the individual child.

Wilson *et al.* (2000) found that carers experienced considerable difficulties in the UK system. They felt that they were often regarded as second-class citizens. Butcher (2005) found in her Australian study that foster carers wanted more support from workers. Similarly, when interviewed, carers in the UK felt that "Sometimes you feel as if you are at the bottom of the pile. Everyone's views (child's/parents/social workers [sic]) seem to come first and you have no say" (Fisher *et al.* 2000: 228). Nutt (2006) conducted an English study into the world views of foster carers and found that there was support for the principle that workers could learn from the expertise of carers, rather than expertise always being seen as flowing in a hierarchical way from workers to carers.

Carers can also experience considerable difficulty when allegations of abuse or poor care standards are made against them.

> Our family felt very betrayed by Social Services' apparent lack of support when allegations were made. When they proved unfounded our social worker was very supportive. I will never get over the feeling of betrayal and after so many years of working together there was not one hint from anyone that they felt it was a mistake or unfounded.
>
> (Fisher *et al.* 2000: 227)

Attrition of trained foster carers has a complex web of causes and is a problem in many places around the world (Bath 2000). Ensuring some stability of the pool of foster carers benefits children. Multiple failed placements for children can have devastating consequences for their life outcomes and is a profound indictment on our current arrangements (Pecora *et al.* 2003, 2005; Osborn and Delfabbro 2006).

There are palpable difficulties for foster carers around the issue of attachment to children in care, and this finding is borne out by the work undertaken by Thorpe and Westerhuis (2006). On the one hand, it is clearly essential that carers can, and should, form relationships with children and young people as foster care is family care designed to nurture children. However, carers need support around decisions for children and young people that do not involve permanent placement with the carer's own family. Unfortunately, too often this issue is ignored or down-played by practitioners. This complex area has no easy solutions.

There are difficulties for carers when decisions are made about care plans for children without their involvement. Many carers have identified issues that they feel have not been taken into consideration and that their own perspectives can be a helpful addition to the whole picture for a child in their care. Carers have also stated that, on occasion, the impact on them of stressful interactions with parents is not acknowledged or is minimized:

> We have experienced threats of serious violence against us and this child from natural parents with previous convictions of serious violence including murder . . . In these circumstances . . . we don't think it appropriate for natural families to know the name or address of the people caring for the child.
>
> (Wilson *et al.* 2000: 201)

An innovative approach in France (International Movement ATD Fourth World 2004), which valued the importance of understanding foster carers' own backgrounds involved helping female foster carers (there was no mention of male carers or partners of female carers) to work with children in their care and understand their families and past events. The innovation came with the decision to start with carers themselves and their own life histories in a positive way, which helped carers feel valued, respected, and listened to, and helped them with their struggles around the family histories of children and young people in care. This relationship-rich approach appears to have had many benefits for children and young people. The joint evaluation by the women who participated found:

> This work gave us a reason to talk with children about their natural family, and to reposition ourselves in relation to that family by reassuring them about our intentions and by demonstrating to them that we weren't trying to replace them.
>
> (International Movement ATD
> Fourth World 2004: 141)

Along with the importance of understanding the experiences of fathers caught up with child protection systems is the need to understand important dimensions of the male foster carer experience. Wilson *et al.* (2007) interviewed men about a range of issues, including their motivations to foster, in a study that highlighted the distinctive and positive contribution of men as foster carers. One participant stated: "I just thought, as a man, you could offer a safe and secure home to that child, as a new role model, which may help them change what they know, or what they think, about men" (Wilson *et al.* 2007: 25).

Foster carers are in a particularly difficult position. There is much rhetoric around partnership with carers which is frequently not realized due to systemic reasons. In a child protection system characterized by anxiety (Munro 1999b) and risk aversion (Webb 2006), children and young people are often removed from their families without the solid investment in working with the family that could lead to changed outcomes in safety and well-being. In many jurisdictions, placement options are limited, with the emergence over recent times, of foster care as the major form of out-of-home care (Maluccio *et al.* 2000). Children are then placed with people who frequently have their own struggles around conceptualizing and coming to terms with their own needs as self-actualized beings beyond the roles they perform in care-giving. Children in care are often traumatized and distressed by the events that led to them coming into care, and almost always by the separation and disruption of leaving their families, even in situations where removal is clearly the only reasonable course of action (Thomson and Thorpe 2004). Children can then be very wary of the best intentioned ministrations of carers. Overlaid over the complex motivations of carers and the deep distress of vulnerable children, the bureaucratized nature of child protection imposes clumsy barriers on best practice outcomes for children.

Foster carer's own children

Another group of interest in foster care narratives are the foster carers' own children. We suggest that the inclusion of the voices of foster carers' children is imperative to a reshaped child protection system and more work in this area is needed. By and large, studies into how fostering is experienced by the children of people who choose to foster (Spears and Cross 2003; Nutt 2006) do not reveal a positive story. In a Swedish study of the children of foster carers Hojer (2007) found that the constraints imposed on family life by the parental decision to undertake fostering were considerable. Many of the children and young people interviewed stated that they had frequently not talked to their parents (or indeed anyone) about their own struggles and issues, as they were aware of the burdens of fostering for their parents. However, the burden carried by children of foster carers was also considerable, and it must be said, invariably without having made the choice themselves to take a foster child or children into the family.

She pulled my hair, so tufts of hair came off. She hit me, called me ugly names, and hid my best things . . . She destroyed the things I loved the most, and hurt me, both physically and mentally. I can't love her. She has hurt me too much.

(Hojer 2007: 78)

Child protection practitioners

Child protection practitioners experience many difficulties working in these systems. Perhaps the well documented problems in recruitment and retention of foster carers (Brown and Bednar 2006) are mirrored in the common experience of workers who find their organizations unsupportive and ready to scapegoat them when problems arise? It is important to avoid the generalization that the experiences of service users and practitioners are the same, but it is also important to acknowledge that both groups are stakeholders. The facts speak for themselves in relation to the constant exodus of workers from child protection agencies, related to the systemic issues identified in Chapter 4.

Workers are vulnerable to being scapegoated unless politicians, bureaucrats and the general public acknowledge and respect the uncertainty and difficulties inherent in working within contested relationships where there are differing perspectives on the issues which have led children to be in need of protection by the state (Ruch 2005). For example, there is an urgent need to acknowledge the difficulties for workers of simultaneously supporting children and young people in care, parents, and foster carers. Indeed, it may be impossible for many workers to successfully remain impartial and non-aligned in current child protection systems, which often have blaming and punitive discourses, and organizational missions that are too broad and all embracing. There needs to be greater recognition of workers' stresses and greater emphasis on addressing it through reflective professional supervision (Ellis 2000; Cooper 2002).

Such recognition would also include an awareness of the formal and informal power relationships between workers and foster carers. That world views and understandings are experienced very differently by workers and parents is clearly illustrated by Holland (2000) who studied their interactions during child protection assessments. She found considerable misunderstandings existed on many levels.

She can't stay after contact tomorrow because she's looking after her sister's kids. (laughs). That's more of a priority! I feel like I'm running around after her all the time and I don't think that's how it should be. She doesn't seem to see how important this could be for her. It's as if she'll fit it in if there's nothing more important to do.

(Holland 2000: 153)

From a relationship perspective, there is potential to reframe this mother's decision positively. Her commitment to caring for children, and to helping her own extended family and the cousins of her own children, could be seen as a sign of strength in her ability to parent. The fact that workers are paid to engage with parents in the interests of children could be seen as a positive, allowing the worker to make the extra effort and cope with differing circumstances to progress decisions about the care of this mother's own children in the context of her broader location in an extended family, thereby building cohesion in the family to which her children belong.

Morris (2005) provides an account of the narratives that operate for workers who stay in beleaguered and under-resourced child protection systems. She used twenty autobiographical essays to explore the willingness of many workers to continue in systems that are widely perceived to be dysfunctional and which, at the very least, do not serve their own best interests. She employed the use of an understanding of counter stories, juxtaposed against master narratives within a feminist inquiry, to argue that the work does confer meaning for many workers.

> I thoroughly enjoy working with children and families and I believed that if I could save one child or family in my career then I would be considered successful in what I was doing and ultimately in making a difference in society.
>
> (Morris 2005: 141)

Callahan's and Lumb's (1995) study captured some worker's comments which were insightful about their roles. They provided accounts which acknowledge the complexity and paradoxes in child protection work and the need for a high level of awareness by workers. "A worker's role is almost as important as the abuser, as we can contribute to the abuse continuing" (Callahan and Lumb 1995: 806). Some workers are also very aware of the power they hold: "I have become more aware of how fearful people are of us . . . It had a real impact on me" (Callahan and Lumb 1995: 807).

It is unsurprising that the experiences of workers in troubled and overloaded child protection systems are, by and large, not positive ones. A small-scale Australian study found that workers felt overwhelmed and besieged (Thomson 2007). The workers in this study demonstrated a high degree of commitment to the children and young people for whom they felt responsible, and this shaped their perceptions of the capability and effectiveness of individual foster carers. This over-arching study finding was strongly positive but this commitment in the face of constraints brought about by high work loads caused considerable stress for workers. "I feel like I am not doing enough for these children . . . it's brought me down . . . (and I have been) angry with myself because I wasn't able to do everything that I wanted to do" (Thomson 2007: 340).

These child protection workers felt uncomfortable when parents and carers asked them for support because they mainly saw themselves as working for the child in care, and did not see it as their role to support others.

The workers experienced some role dissonance, as they found it difficult to balance competing demands on them from children and young people, from parents and from carers.

> A lotta things they expect the worker to do, I don't have the capacity to do. I just can't do it you know ... but ... the first thing they do is just say well ring the worker and if there is a problem bang, you're it and then if there's a target, you're it as well.
>
> (Thomson 2007: 343)

We now turn to examine the perspectives of other stakeholders in child protection systems, particularly those who are community-based representatives. The complex issues that they face are important to address if substantive systemic reform is to be achieved. These stakeholders are centrally located in shaping the types of responses and interventions that meet families' and parents' needs, and which provide the most effective sorts of protection for children from, and prevention of, abuse and neglect, particularly in impoverished communities and neighborhoods.

Community stakeholders

The delivery of child protection and/or child welfare services involves multiple stakeholders, all of them potentially holding competing theoretical positions and a wide range of approaches to the needs of children and families, service priorities, assessment processes, risk measures, and performance and outcome measures. Spokespersons for different views and concerns about child protection all compete for attention in the "marketplace" of this important public policy issue. They often represent different "camps" which hold significantly different opinions about moral, political, as well as empirical arguments about the nature of the problems as well as the options for solutions.

The stakeholders to which we refer include, non-government and community organizations, self-help groups, educators and researchers, journalists (often referred to simply as "the media"), survivors of abuse, "claimant advocates," or "accused advocates" (Mildred 2003), professional associations, politicians and political parties, and population groups such as Indigenous and culturally and linguistically diverse communities. Clearly, not all the views of all of these stakeholders are at odds—as Mildred says, there are some "strange bedfellows" (Mildred 2003: 493) in the shifting camps—nor can all views be incorporated into policy frameworks at any one time. Each wields differential authority and exerts different influence depending on personal charisma, as well as the idiosyncrasies of the cultural, political and societal context in which they represent themselves. They may well be and often are, in competition as they vie for public opinion about the problems and the solutions. Sadly, the contest for public attention generally occurs after one or more tragic events have occurred that involves death or injury to a child, which in turn lead to community distress and outrage, and an urgent need for government to be seen to be "doing something."

All of these competing theoretical positions and approaches are influenced by the experiences, values, morality, and beliefs of their proponents as well as the cultural and institutional contexts in which they are expressed (Freymond and Cameron 2006). The theoretical issues and questions include the following:

1   The standard of care that should be expected of parents: Is there a universal standard that should be used to judge all parents? If not, how does one mediate different standards for different individuals and communities?
2   The role of the state: At what point, with what amount of justification, and under whose authorization can the state intervene in family life?
3   The competing rights of children and parents: The simplest question here is; which rights should dominate, under what conditions?
4   The best interests of the child: What does this mean in context and how is such a judgment made "over time"?
5   The rights of a child to the retention of family connection versus permanent placement or adoption: When, if at all, must the right of a child to her/his connection with family be sacrificed for his/her safety?
6   The role of primary, secondary or tertiary prevention: A key question here that is often presented is—does prevention work in the protection of vulnerable children?
7   Treatment and punishment: Should parents who fail in their duty to children be punished or assisted to provide better care—or both?
8   Long-term or short-term interventions: If the aim is to assist parents, how much support should they get, for how long, and from whom (NGO or statutory authority)?
9   The incidence of reporting of child abuse: The key questions here are about the differences between numbers of reports and incidence of "abuse." Does the vast increase in numbers of reported children in Anglophone countries represent a diagnostic inflation or actual increases in harms to children?
10 Evidence about effectiveness of interventions: Questions here focus not only on what interventions help children and families, but which service providers are best equipped to provide these services, for example, non-government or statutory providers?

These competing voices are in competition for at least one or all of the following: validation of their own positions; the influence of public policy and decision making; and funding. And, when they compete in the highly emotional environment in which they do, it is at least arguable that the ones that are heard are those whose message is most likely to sway the public and the government of the day—with or without evidence to substantiate their claims.

The relatively recent research of Jane Mildred (2003) in the US is interesting in relation to the competing claims of various stakeholders in the child protection arena. While the focus was on competing claims about sexual abuse, her research is relevant to the generic work of child protection. She interviewed forty "opinion leaders" who were viewed to have brought claims about child sexual abuse to the attention of people in the Western world. Her very thorough analysis outlines a continuum of "claimsmaking" which, she argues, demonstrates that different views do not represent scientifically validated positions or evidence but, rather, they reflect often acrimonious disputes based on differences in moral positions and attitudes, family experience, gender and persuasion. It is interesting to note that she found no correlation between the various "claims camps" and political stance. She says:

> Therefore some child sexual abuse conflicts may be inevitable, and to a certain extent unresolvable, because they reflect what the issue symbolizes as much as, or more than, they reflect actual differences of opinion about issues related to child sexual abuse.
>
> (Mildred 2003: 502)

Most importantly, and of relevance to the argument in this book and chapter, Mildred (2003) goes on to say that "there is reason to be concerned about the lack of constructive communication within and among the constituencies involved in conflicts around child sexual abuse" (p. 502). What is already apparent is that there are a large number of reasons why some "claim makers" or stakeholders may be more excluded than others from influencing policy and practice. Some of these reasons are as follows:

*   There has been urgency among many "claimsmakers" to establish the facts about the vulnerability of children and the reality of child abuse to a disbelieving and perhaps complacent public. Powerful media images of injured children, stories of terrible tragedies involving children, and heart-rending narratives by survivors of abuse and their advocates, provide a clear pathway to action—even though the outcomes of such action can only be surmised to be positive.
*   The dramatic increase in scholarship about child protection over the last 30 years has placed ever-increasing emphasis on expert opinion and expertise in the management of Anglophone child protection systems. An expert model is now in evidence and this is likely to have a rocky relationship, at best, with any community voice that attempts to portray any other view that is not informed by research. Of course, the status of professional expertise remains strong despite the fact that this scholarship is itself full of contested perspectives and demonstrates that there are no perfect working models of child protection.
*   The perspectives of parents, children and young people, and adults who have experienced the care system and those who work in such systems,

have increasingly been the subject of research. However, their ability to influence the juggernaut that has developed appear to be limited, as political and institutional systems become increasingly bureaucratized in the face of anxieties and fears about child deaths and injuries. Nowhere is this more evident than in the longstanding, vocal, and increasingly well researched, views of Indigenous people whose powerlessness, despite their manifest voice, is palpable as they witness the increasing numbers of their children being taken into state care.

• It is also evident in the difficulty that statutory child protection systems appear to have in working in partnership and trust with non-government and community-based organizations that aim to assist families in need but are generally so poorly resourced to do so.

What is very apparent is that the result of these competing claims and the power differentials that surround them is that they all battle for a voice against an increasingly risk-averse and proceduralized institutional structure. A commitment to overcoming the adversarial nature of relationships to be found in the contemporary highly proceduralized and legalistic child protection systems is crucial in bringing about reform, but is not necessarily welcomed by governments under pressure to "fix" child protection and punish errant parents.

Summary

We suggest that the inclusion of children, parents, community organizations, and other stakeholders must be the hallmark of a reformed and caring system. We take the position that highly proceduralized, low-risk threshold approaches to the safety and well-being of very vulnerable children and young people are not working. In the UK, the approach has extended to the high-level surveillance of family life entailed in tracking methodologies (Parton 2006a).

While there are difficulties in the service user and community stakeholder framework which seeks to challenge the increasingly hierarchical approach to the protection of children, we suggest that change is both imperative and possible. Embracing a more inclusive framework is not a new conceptualization: these concepts were developed by Beresford and Croft in a number of publications (1980, 1993, 2004). Holman (1993) has been another long-term visionary in promoting an emancipatory framework that involves service users at all levels, and challenges the underlying disadvantage that leads people to service user status and allows divisions based on social position to continue.

In relation to foster carers, the concept of partnership promoted here also sits well with the needs of carers in a revamped child protection system. Many carers have suffered from being conceptualized as services users within a professionalized discourse with one central actor—a professional child protection practitioner. To date, attempts at partnership have often been clumsy, but in our view, there is considerable scope to develop further in this area. The model of exclusive fostering in some jurisdictions has largely failed and there needs to be a wholehearted commitment to a new approach to partnership.

In relation to practitioners, new approaches need to embrace the multiple demands and difficulties fundamental to effective management of the role of a child protection practitioner, through the provision of mentoring, role modeling, and supportive supervision by senior staff. The failure to provide professional supervision often results in workers feeling isolated and compelled to develop their own models of practice, potentially with an absence of direction and in an atheoretical way.

However difficult it may be, it is imperative that the views of a much broader range of stakeholders are considered if policy makers and governments are to learn from what works for different cohorts of children and young people, in different environments and communities, in other jurisdictions and in contexts other than the Anglophone countries. All child protection and child welfare systems are said to have weaknesses as well as strengths. The one strength that Anglophone countries do have is that they have managed to convince the public that there is a need to safeguard children and keep them safe. We need to maximize this strength by attending very closely to the diverse voices that can inform policy and practice and reduce the iatrogenesis for children, parents, families, and communities caught up in our contemporary child protection orthodoxy and arrangements.

In the next chapter we place the discussion about stakeholders and "claims-makers" within the much broader debate about what we describe as the reforms that are required if we are to address the problems and meet the challenges that we have enunciated in this first section of the book. We now turn to our proposals for fundamental reforms, which address a range of issues at the organizational, program, and practice levels in order to change the nature of the social relations that are central to our societal efforts to protect children and young people and prevent abuse and neglect.

Part III

A child and family well-being reform agenda

> The difficulty is not finding new ways of doing things, but in letting go of the old ways of doing things.
>
> Maynard Keynes

6 Reforming child protection
Principles and processes

In the previous chapters we identified key themes in the failure of child protection systems in Anglophone countries to move the spotlight of policy and
practice away from a narrow focus on child protection to one which is much
more concerned with early intervention and the improvement of children's
well-being. Central to our argument about change are two premises:

1   improving policy and practice must recognize the crucial ethical and moral
    dimensions to the work; and
2   reform which concentrates on modification of technical systems is quite
    inadequate.

Modifications that have incorporated broadening the scope of prevention
while at the same time trying to reduce the chances of a child dying have
put ever greater emphasis upon introducing complex systems, intricate procedures, risk assessments, relentless monitoring and a preoccupation with the
management of risk. Further, there has been increased curbing of professional
discretion along with the expectation that front-line child protection practitioners follow exhaustive and complex procedural and ever more legalistic
guidance. What has emerged is a child welfare system that is complicit in
racism and the depoliticization of its activities, and which can well be accused
of dismantling the social networks in civil society in general, but in Black
and Indigenous communities in particular (Roberts 2002: vii). These increasingly modified systems are antithetical to the requirement of work in complex
family and community relationships—work which demands a capacity for
tolerance of uncertainty, and creative practice in order to undertake in-depth
assessments and formulate professional partnerships *with* children, young
people, parents, families, and communities. To repeat what Howe said over
10 years ago, a number of these changes "substitute confidence in systems
for trust in individual professionals" (Howe 1996: 92). It is now very clear
that modifying the current framework is not working. Even the significant
modification of trying to differentiate cases between "child in need of support"
("child concern report") and child in need of protection ("child maltreatment
allegation") has not worked.

In this chapter we provide an overview of the reforms required to address what we assert are fundamental and serious flaws in contemporary child protection practice in Anglophone countries—flaws that are more than simply organizational and practice ones that can be remedied with procedural changes, reparative work, and new procedures, diagrams, and flow charts We have already argued that these defects reside in the very essence of the philosophical underpinnings of the way child protection is conceptualized and framed in Anglophone countries.

We are very aware that we are not alone in this view. Multiple scholars and practitioners across the continents have been urging serious change for the last few years (Roberts 2002; Lombardi 2003; Prilleltensky and Prilleltensky 2006; Parton 2006a). A particularly blunt statement to this effect is made by Berg and Kelly in the introductory pages of their book: "It is no secret . . . the universal opinion is that the system is broken and something needs to be done to fix it. However, most people have no comprehensive ideas on how to "fix" the problem" (Berg and Kelly 2000: 3). On the same issue but more recently, David Stoez (2007) puts his position very clearly alongside a firm recommendation: "Child protective services is irreparably broken and should be replaced by a new infrastructure that assures vulnerable children and troubled families the services they need" (Stoez 2007: 224).

A comprehensive new approach

We concur with these and many other writers who suggest that the problem is no longer one that can be fixed by tinkering with the system at the edges to "tidy it up." A corollary to this argument is that we propose a fundamental revision of policies and practices that is characterized by:

- radical rethinking about what we mean by the terms "harm," "abuse," "child safety," and "child protection";
- a foundation plank of relevant evidence about what constitutes the sort of severity that requires reporting or referral to a forensic, investigative, statutory child protection system (which must be the referral place of "last resort" for children and families in need but the first portal for children in real danger);
- a clear and unwavering focus on positive outcomes for children and families as the central goal of a dynamic system that promotes the well-being of children and their parents, families, and communities;
- a child-centered, family-focused, culturally respectful framework for intervention; and
- ethical, value-driven and relationship-based practice that is grounded in, and facilitative of, neighborhood- and community-based social care systems.

Central to our proposals about the need to develop a comprehensive new approach rather than continuing to pursue the policy of "incremental creep," is our acceptance of Giddens' proposition that expert systems—such as the child protection one—fail as a result of "design faults" in the system rather than simply due to the failure of the "operators" of those systems (Giddens 1990). These design faults are not operational ones, but exist in the way that need and clients and services are understood, and in how meaning is constructed about children, parents, families, safety, and abuse. The evidence for the seriousness of the design faults is manifest in the research that has been outlined in previous chapters, which clearly shows that at every level the elements of the child protection system that has developed in Anglophone countries in recent times are failing—children are suffering, families are fracturing, communities are reeling, staff are turning over faster than they can be trained and inducted, and taxpayers are paying more and more for child protection services with no proven efficacy in many instances. Fragmented remedies based on one-dimensional revisions will not alter the system failures. A comprehensive revision of principles, policies and practices is required and a new conceptual framework that values the lived experience of children, their families, and their communities must be developed.

The need for such a new framework has challenged our colleagues in other areas of human service endeavor, such as mental health services, across the world in recent times (Turnell and Edwards 1999; Berg and Kelly 2000; Hutchinson and Sudia 2002; Stanley *et al.* 2003). In the words of the Berg and Kelly:

> The field of mental health is undergoing a re-examination of how services are delivered, who delivers them, and what the results are . . . The result is a nagging feeling that there is something missing in the expert driven medical model . . . The new thrust has come from the culture of empowerment, the desire of professionals to work with the client in an egalitarian, democratic manner that respects and values a client's individual views and way of being in the world.
>
> (Berg and Kelly 2000: 16)

And most powerfully, they assert:

> We believe that it is time for those in CPS and the child welfare field to institutionalize the paradigm based on respect and empowerment . . . This new approach encourages the worker to see the client as a repository of resources, not a pool of pathology.
>
> (Berg and Kelly 2000: 16)

Beyond risk and child death

In outlining our comprehensive new approach, we repeat "the unspeakable" and consider the significance of the policy premise and apparent public conviction that we can develop systems that can ensure that no child will die. We also reflect on the implicit, if not explicit, and growing public expectation that we have a moral obligation to ensure that every child must realize her or his maximum potential (however this is measured)—as if this idea is unproblematic and the ideal can be achieved without compromising other aspects of that child's life or the lives of her/his family and community. In referring to the contentious issue of preventing all child deaths and the unrealistic expectation that any system can guarantee safety to all children, we do not aim to diminish the significance of the goal of providing safety for children. What we assert is what appears to be unpalatable and this is that the means we have adopted to ensure the safety of children in Anglophone countries may well be an illusion, which, while of noble intent, is producing more harm than good.

We are not only failing to realize our child safety goals in many instances but we are using means and mechanisms to achieve these goals that are counterproductive to the interests of vast numbers of children, their families and their communities—and ultimately of civil society itself. If this level of iatrogenesis was detected in any other area such as health services, there is no doubt that dramatic changes would be demanded and made. Arguably, even children most in need of the extreme form of protective service that requires removing them from parents and family, are ill served in a system that is overwhelmed with referrals for families in need, and unable to focus on providing them with the level of care that attempts to remediate their already significant and "unearned" disadvantage.

In saying this, we continue to affirm that we need a system that:

- directly attends to the needs of children, intervenes well to protect and provide the highest quality alternative for children and young people who really cannot be cared for by their birth parents;
- builds capacity of families and communities; recognizes systemic complexity and the multiple pathways that lead to the physical and/or psychological harm of children;
- is focused on early intervention and prevention;
- integrates services across government, non government and community; and
- is based on core ethical principles and values of respect and justice as well as duty.

It needs to be noted that we approach child protection very broadly and locate child protection systems within a contemporary understanding of what a humane civil society might look like—one in which a commitment to maximizing child and family well-being rather than risk-aversion must be a central platform.

And to again speak the unspeakable—whatever we do there always will be the risk and reality of child deaths. Ferguson's important question, in his book,

Protecting Children in Time (2004) is "how has the powerful idea that we can protect all children developed?" He states, "it is remarkable how little attention has been given to a full sociological interrogation of this ideal" (p. 3). His examination of the history and current status of that endeavor is compelling reading and talks to the urgent need to rethink "the global idea and ideal of child protection" (Ferguson 2004: 3) and its associated attributions of responsibility to human agency when the ideal fails, and to also attend instead to both the "design faults" that Giddens proposes, and the "complex nature of human agency" which ensures that simple service responses will never address the complexity of family life and distress (Ferguson 2004: 196).

Despite our best intentions, it may well be that not all child deaths can or ever will be avoided. And indeed, it is at least possible if not highly likely that the more risk-dominated child protection policies focus on widening the reporting net to include more and more reporters and indicators of risk (from poor diet to poor hygiene), the more likely it is that we actually increase the danger for those most likely to suffer serious harm because we are distracted by the avalanche of concerns raised about poor parenting rather than dangerous families (Hood *et al.* 2001). In this light, it was disturbing to hear this pronouncement by a presenter at the Ninth Australasian Conference on Child Abuse and Neglect (2003)—a pronouncement that went publicly unchallenged. A presenter said "there is no such thing as an accidental injury; there is only supervisory neglect." In other words, if any child is injured or harmed, it could have been prevented, someone is at fault, and someone must be punished.

The framework from which we need to move is one explicitly driven by profoundly provocative images of children being rescued from failing, bad, and cruel parents and being placed in the hands of a bounteous state which, acting as the new parent (or grandparent) provides a wholesome remedy and permanent alternative. While this is not the image held by most practitioners, scholars, agency managers or academics most of whom are fully aware of the limitations of the current forensically charged system in Anglophone countries, it seems likely that it is the image held by the general public and, of course, the media who want to believe it to be true and who drive the public and political responses as they fulfill their primary aim, which is sell stories and advertising to an ever-anxious society.

The centrality of the family

In this idealized world of child protective services that is constructed and is implicitly, if not explicitly, manifest in much public policy, every child is expected to achieve her/his maximum potential, no child will die, and if a parent is seen to fail (by whatever the articulated or unarticulated standard of the time), they will be punished and their child(ren) will be placed in the safe care of foster parents who are patiently waiting in the wings to embrace and nurture them. Even if there was an endless supply of taxpayer funding available to fulfill this fantasy, and an endless supply of carers, the idealized image is seriously flawed for a number of reasons. However, one dominates all and that is one represented by the dictum—"family is family forever"—or, in the words of Schneider, "they are yours and they stay with you as you stay with them" (quoted in Penglase 2005: 272). A particularly poignant variation of this dictum is a phrase used in the Solomon Islands to signify the unity of family and humanity, "Me Belong You—You Belong Me." Whatever the view of well-meaning adults, professionals, the media and politicians, children and adults who were in the "care system" are telling us that fundamental to life, let alone quality, is connection with family, and that the loss of family is one of the most traumatizing of any childhood event wherever one lives in the world.

This idea is most poignantly expressed by young people in a very recent study, conducted by researchers at the Australian Institute of Family Studies who undertook interviews with Indigenous young people in care, professionals from government, non-government, and Indigenous agencies, and carers of Aboriginal and Torres Strait Islander children. The headline for one particular section of their report which records what young people say about their experience of out-of-home care holds these haunting words:

> Q: If there was one thing in your lives that you could change, what would it be?
> A: We would really, really want to be with our parents.
>
> (Higgins *et al.* 2007: 1)

What these researchers say in their reports is salutary and complex, but the core is well expressed in this very simple summary from the report:

> The messages from the young people in this study focused almost exclusively on the importance to them of maintaining connections to their family, their community and their culture. The overriding message from young people was that they wanted to go home to their families. This is an important reminder that although the safety of children and young people is of paramount importance, it is not the only issue to be considered in securing the best interests of the child.
>
> (*Ibid.*: 9)

The emerging realization of the devastation that is subsequent to the loss of family is testimony to the ubiquitous failure of an adult-centered approach to the interpretation of the "best interests" of the child that is implicit in much of the research with children, and is but one of the pointers to the failure of the child protection paradigm we have followed for the last 20 or so years.

A new approach to evidence

Practitioners and policy makers in most Anglophone countries have to manage the history of child removal that was motivated by ideals rather than evidence. Fundamental to these ideals was the commendable intention of improving the welfare of children, but this did not include any consultation with the very people whose welfare was at stake. We now know that the result has often been one in which dislocation, trauma, and further abuse has been experienced by these very children who were "saved." The research literature—much of it from adults who are "graduates" of the care system—is replete with evidence of the harm done to many children when well-intentioned people have removed children from the care of their families—even though it may have been done with the "best interests of the child" in mind (Parton *et al.* 1997).

Two particular policies of many that highlight the dangers of well-intentioned, evidence-free practice are the forced emigration of child migrants from the UK to Canada and Australia, and the removal of Indigenous children in various parts of the world (Fournier and Crey 1997; National Inquiry into the Separation of Aboriginal and Torres Strait Islander Children from their Families 1997). Both policies claimed to focus on meeting the needs of vulnerable children. This history represents the extreme of conceptualization of child welfare policies and practices that privileged one perspective of a child's best interests, denied cultural diversity in child rearing practices, and justified a violent means (child removal) by arguing for a greater good (integration into another culture). Very important historical lessons from these periods of child care policy contribute to our thinking in this chapter. The story of the transport of unaccompanied child migrants from the United Kingdom to Canada and Australia in the interests of a "good future" and settling the colonies with "British stock" is one that still shocks us (Bean and Melville 1989; Australian Senate Community Affairs References Committee 2001a, b) and led one scholar to write:

> It is hoped that the story—for many a tragic story—of the British child migrants to Australia will provide some lessons for the future. One is that any government or private organization must think long and hard before it separates children from their parents, families and cultural heritage. If it is ever the correct thing to do it must be a measure of last resort.
>
> (Buti 2002: 1)

The faulty premise about the apparent inconsequentiality of family in the lives of children is but one aspect of the absence of an adequate evidential basis for the interventions in the lives of children and families that have been justified in the name of child protection. Research with Indigenous communities across the world should be sufficient to show us how catastrophic is the result of this premise. In relation to this, it is useful to read one of the most profound statements in the recent far reaching review of the child and family welfare system in Manitoba, Canada: "[The] protection based model of child welfare has not worked for Aboriginal people in the past and it cannot work now" (Hardy *et al.* 2006: 27).

And this powerful comment should not only be applied to the fate of Aboriginal children at the hands of our well-intentioned child protection programs. It applies equally strongly to all racial minority groups and has been powerfully portrayed by Roberts (2002) in her book *Shattered Bonds: The Color of Child Welfare*.

If we need evidence of how widespread is the iatrogenesis in our contemporary child protection paradigm, salutary reading is provided by the Australian Senate Community Affairs References Committee (2005) in the Senate Report *Protecting vulnerable children: A national challenge, Second Report on the inquiry into children in institutional care*. It is estimated that 500,000 adults in Australia once lived in the care system. Their submissions and stories are harrowing and talk not just to the abuses that occurred in the care system but to the total failure of past and present policies to appreciate the priority need of children to connection with family and culture. One of the survivors of this system is Joanna Penglase (2005) whose book based on her own experience and doctoral research is titled *Orphans of the Living*. In this book, the evocative title of which tells its story of loss so powerfully, she has this to say: "We effectively treated our most vulnerable children as criminals when their only crime was the deprivation of one of the most fundamental of human needs—the love and care of their parents" (Penglase, 2004: back cover).

Let's have some real change for a change

One of the major problems faced by child protection practitioners and colleagues in allied disciplines who want to do things differently, is that despite evidence of gross failure, the existing paradigm continues alongside a relentless "tinkering on the edges." Rather than real change (which, we argue, requires a change of paradigm) what child welfare practitioners generally confront is an escalating patchwork of legislation and a plethora of rules, policies, practices, and procedures that they have to understand and follow under ever-tightening systems of managerial oversight and "quality control," and amidst a discourse that is increasingly dominated by the language of risk, surveillance, blaming, child rescue, and forensic investigation. The increasingly restrictive procedures and well documented risk management protocols that these practitioners face are endemic in Anglophone countries and have generally been introduced in the wake of episodic panics that are generated by individual tragedies and scandals. And escalating reports about the abuse of children and the failure of professionals and governments to stop child deaths or even reduce the incidence of what is called "child abuse" continue to fuel the fear of already anxious communities (Munro 1999b), and lead to relentless retreats to proceduralism that appears disconnected from any debate about either ethics or evidence.

These increasing performance pressures are occurring at a time that the term "child abuse" is being subjected to unremitting definitional inflation as cultural mores, changing expectations and the heightened awareness of the vulnerabilities of childhood, redefine behaviors as harmful and abusive (Mansell 2006a,b). And whatever the emerging vagaries in the definitions of abuse (such as witnessing domestic violence, child obesity and supervisory neglect), professionals and the public are increasingly subject to ever-burgeoning mandatory reporting laws that have produced an avalanche of reports—generally associated with endemic systemic social and family problems—that cannot be assessed let alone responded to (Harries and Clare 2002; Melton 2005; Mansell 2006a,b; D. Scott 2006a).

One major change required is to support rather than monitor families. Arguably, the Anglophone child protection has become obsessed with reporting, investigating, and monitoring. Failure of systems to respond to impossible numbers of reports is feeding a renewed public panic and, as many commentators now observe, child protection practices as we have developed them in the Anglophone world are in meltdown (Ferguson 2004; D. Scott 2006a; Testro and Peltola 2007; Pelton 2008). No amount of money being poured in to investigation of these often mandatory reports is producing measurable benefits for children, parents, families, or communities, let alone ones that justify the expense involved. Children continue to struggle for success in households that have limited resources and/or where their parents or caregivers themselves struggle with various problems that often seem insurmountable. It would appear that many of these children and families are on the "radar" of child protective services, but that rather than receiving assistance to reduce the impact of the stresses they are experiencing, they are "monitored" until the threshold for removal is reached.

A recently released research report on the experiences of parents of children who have been taken into the care of the state provides powerful evidence of the added burden that monitoring without support places on these families (Family Inclusion Network 2007). And evidence for this practice was stated— apparently unashamedly—in a recent media report by a Minister responsible for child welfare in Australia. He is reported to have defended the attempted and foiled removal of two children by saying, "the department had been watching the two families involved and caseworkers acted when the situation worsened." The non-government support worker involved in this case is reported to have responded with, "the state government should provide more funding for local organizations to work with women and children, rather than intervening" (ABC News 2007).

What we see in the example above—and one that is no doubt familiar to workers worldwide—is more than evidence of the absurdity of monitoring family stress. We see that two approaches to the welfare of children and families are in collision—the state-funded system that is monitoring for risk and removing the children when the risk reaches a worker's tolerance threshold, and a community support system with minimal funding trying to ameliorate family distress in order to keep the family together.

Supporting workers

Media images of scapegoats haunt the lives of many dedicated child welfare professionals who come from a range of disciplines. No one wants to be accused of mishandling an assessment of abuse and become the next scape-goat. The people who work in child welfare and child protection are generally driven by a concern for the well-being of children. None of them want a child to suffer any harm. None of them want to deprive a child of his/her family unless it is absolutely necessary and will guarantee the child's well-being. None of them want to be party to the violation of parental and family rights and integrity; and yet there is increasing evidence that parents and families have suffered irrevocable harm due to intrusive child welfare practices (Waldfogel 1998), and practitioners are helpless to change the paradigm because they work in systems that are subservient to politically sensitive governments and managers.

We need to honor those workers who dedicate their lives to children's needs by being clear with the public that the task of ensuring the protection of all children from harm and even death is an impossible one and the job is unremittingly difficult (Neuberger 2005). Unless we do this soon we will see a continuation of the dramatic turnover of staff with the ongoing iatrogenic effects this has on vulnerable children, parents, families and communities. But, as a priority, we need to free social work and child protection practi-tioners from the shackles of "disciplining the poor" (Levitas 1998) by "case managing" poor families and those struggling with mental illness, family violence and substance misuse. We need to give these professionals the capacity and the go-ahead to augment the resources of people who love their children (however inadequately), and enable them to understand and engage with the "life-worlds" of families who are seriously marginalized already in societies that have been easily swayed by political and media focus on the dualisms of deserving and undeserving. And we also need to educate them well enough and support them in their professional judgment so that they can discern the dangerous families who really do pose a risk to their children.

Again, most importantly, we need to reorient the philosophy and guiding principles of child welfare practice and practitioners. We need to return to work that is relationship-based rather than procedurally dominated and "managed." The recognition of the centrality of relationship and connection in the lives of children needs to be mirrored in the way that workers do their work and are supported and encouraged. While evidence-driven understanding of child and family well-being must obviously sit in the forefront of the minds of all workers, their own capacity for building relationships with children and parents must be developed and sustained. We know from the abundant research with families and workers that this is not the paradigm currently informing most Anglophone child protection practice. Indeed, an alternative set of principles dominate—"don't get involved," "don't trust," "watch your back," is what workers often describe.

Moving beyond the rhetoric

It is essential that we change more than the rhetoric, and, as noted by many writers, there has been much rhetoric in the policies and legislation that have littered our child welfare/protection information pathways over the last decade (Buckley 2003). The rhetoric talks of "partnerships," "family participation," increasing input from children, increasing family supports, and many such principles and is well represented in inquiry reports across the world. It has all been said before. There is rarely anything new in inquiries that call for systemic change, and we argue that none of the very laudatory principles that are aired in recommendations following inquiries across the world will change the fundamental problem unless there is a dramatic change of philosophy—one that incorporates so much of what has repeatedly been said by Indigenous people. The real question is not—how do we improve child protection practices? It is worth reiterating the assertion made earlier, that the protection-based model of child welfare has not worked. What we need is a transformative process that moves beyond the old rhetoric and paradigm.

In order to answer the question, "how can we best manage a transformative process to shift the focus of responses to child abuse from a reactive crisis-driven mode to a sustainable whole-of-community approach to the well-being and protection of children?", the Ministerial Council of Child Protection in Western Australia commissioned and then endorsed a comprehensive report which included a model for services that challenged the ideal of modifying the current child protection orthodoxy. Among other things, this report recommended the move to "a whole-of-society approach":

- in which children and young people are on everyone's agenda;
- where children and young people are well represented and properly consulted;
- where there is a well-articulated ethical framework dealing with structure, process and values; and
- where there are high quality and targeted services for children in need of protection or at risk of serious harm.

(Harries *et al.* 2004: 1)

The authors of this report argue that governments must move to implement real change rather than increase the rhetoric and to do so we need to move from a focus on notification of suspected abuse which has caught up many children, young people, and families in a web of chaos (secondary abuse); reduced the capacity of families and communities (US Department of Health & Human Services 1993); distracted us from primary and secondary prevention; and, has produced no hard evidence of efficacy. They suggest that such a system will:

- recognize systemic complexity and the multiple pathways that lead children and families into problems;
- focus on early intervention and prevention;
- be able to intervene when it is clear that it really does need to protect children and young people at real risk; and
- build the capacity of families and communities.

A reorienting of thinking

Of crucial importance, the system we develop must not be driven and serviced by government with non-government services providing only the "padding." In order to capitalize on the urgent need to grow civil society and civic structures that embrace the needs of children and families, this reformed system must be integrated across government, non-government and community. In doing this, we need to re-examine the roles of state, market, family and community in supporting the well-being of all citizens and discard the "othering" notions of western citizenship that so easily establish dualities of "deserving and undeserving people," "bad mothers and good mothers," "vulnerable children or predatory children" and concern themselves with justice toward only those constituted as worthy (Hudson 2003: 183).

We need a reorientation of thinking about what works to keep children safe and foster their well-being; to move from being risk-based and deficit-oriented to strengths- and capacity-centered. We need to accept that we "cannot keep doing it the way we once did" (Stewart-Weeks 2000: 279) and start really investing in a "People Paradigm" rather than "Family Responsibility Paradigm." One way of doing this is to start privileging trust as an essential and precious ingredient of civil society and one that is easily corroded by reporting and surveillance systems. We need to reduce inter-agency barriers to communication and develop our capacity again to meet local needs.

One of the major challenges is how to re-engage ordinary citizens, generally called the community, in the deliberations about how we are to provide the sort of care that children, young people and families need—but particularly those who are not gifted with resource advantages, whether these be financial, psychological or physical. To do this we need the media to assist us to facilitate community awareness about the distinction between the relatively rare incidents of child cruelty/abuse produced by pathological individuals, and child neglect and harm that is often the product of systemic forces such as poverty, illness, and family and community violence. We need to be honest about the fact that the only way possible to protect every child from all harm and injury at home is to have a surveillance system that monitors families 24 hours per day and thus surrender our hard-won civil rights to the state.

The media is often accused of increasing moral panics about child abuse. Conversely, we wonder how much it is used by people with an interest in generating such panics, or simply by those well-intentioned people who have wanted to highlight the real and ongoing vulnerability of children. We reiterate that we do not wish to vilify the media and hold it responsible for dangerous practices. Practices are dangerous because workers do get it wrong and when this happens it is important that they are held accountable. The media has an important role to play in highlighting public concerns and it is indeed responsible for informing the public.

An interesting recommendation from a recent Canadian report from Manitoba involves acknowledging and anticipating the need for media involvement "when the media's legitimate focus is not on a crisis or tragedy" (Hardy *et al.* 2006: 22). The authors recommend "annually inviting the media to an information session to fully explain how the system works and how decisions are made, and to answer their questions about the system, unrelated to any case" (Hardy *et al.* 2006: 22). This is, in our view, a great start albeit that it takes a minimalist position on a most serious issue—that of increasing public awareness. The media is a pivotal partner in informing community attitudes about the need for systems of care that work for children, families, and communities. The public must know what researchers and scholars now know—that the systems we have established to protect and care for children are failing not because of worker or system malfunction (although it is inevitable that as with all human endeavors there will be some cases of negligence), but because of the fundamental design faults that start with the very premises of Anglophone child protection policies and practices.

In terms of organizational structures, we need to develop new ways of thinking about the continuum of care and control and realign policy frameworks to better balance social care and social control outcomes. One way forward, we argue, is to separate the investigatory and helping functions to increase focus on the different core missions of both of these. Importantly, we need a separate organization to specifically address the high level of need of children in care and ensure their connection with family and community is sustained.

The centrality of neighborhoods and community-based services

We need to encourage supportive neighborhoods rather than promote fear and encourage retribution and punishment for any parent who is seen to fail what are often culturally dictated standards of care rather than breaches of criminal codes. And we need to strengthen neighborhoods rather than encourage an ongoing fortress mentality in which those who have most can lock themselves away from the sights and needs of those who have less. To do this, policy makers and legislators as well as practitioners need to engage the media in courageous debates about the reality of what is possible in caring for and protecting children.

Support for children and families who are struggling with systemic disadvantages such as poverty, ill health, forced migration, and family violence is not achieved with quick fix solutions. There needs to be a longer-term focus to assistance. Such assistance cannot be "delivered" by child protection agencies that are expert-based, distant and residual in their purpose. Instead, such assistance needs to come from people being part of the fabric of neighborhood and community that sustains their children and their families and in so doing, builds communities, social capital, and civil societies that in turn grow their own capacity to care for children.

Such a model sits in stark contract to the gloomy image painted by Robert Putnam (2000) in *Bowling Alone,* his groundbreaking work on the loss of community spirit and social capital in America and implications of this for the American social fabric. And, he asserts, the impact of the loss of community and social capital on the lives of children and families has been profound. He states: "social capital is second only to poverty in the breadth and depth of its effects on children's lives" (Putnam 2000: 297). He shows how loss of community correlates with rises in all of the ills that are associated with high levels of trauma and low levels of safety—abuse, suicide, homicide, criminality, and violence. Potently, he observes from his research that "child abuse rates are higher where neighborhood cohesion is lower" (Putnam 2000: 298).

Joan Lombardi, who has dedicated her life to the development of systems of child care in the United States, is deeply concerned with the loss of supports for communities that have followed ambivalent public policies about social changes and the role of mothers, fathers and families. She outlines a comprehensive and, she argues, time-tested and workable strategy for regrowth of community for children in her book, *Time to Care: Redesigning Child Care* (2003). She uses the metaphor of a child-care quilt—and says that such a quilt is made up of "a community support system for parents and providers," "encourages citizen participation," and "in the process brings together the young and the old to create new extended families" (Lombardi 2003: 129). This strategy, she suggests, is like all of the ones that promote community, and is based on the now extensive research knowledge such as that outlined by Putnam, that children thrive where communities (rather than child protection teams) flourish. She talks of the importance of "networks," of building "gateways", of building "platforms" that "stand ready" to "help children and their families" (Lombardi 2003: 130).

It is pertinent at this stage to remind ourselves that the implementation of these ideas will not be simple, and, along with auspicious scholars such as Melton *et al.* (2002) we acknowledge the hard task ahead in doing things differently. In their far-reaching report *Toward a Child-Centered Neighborhood-Based Child Protection System,* these authors address the vital and urgent need to regenerate neighborhoods in order to foster child well-being and safety. In particular, they enunciate carefully the challenges we all face in re-creating caring communities that ensure that child protection is simply a "part of every day life" (2002: 263). Small *et al.* (2002), writing in this same report, say, "the structural changes needed at every level to ensure child safety pose formidable challenges." They offer an additional note of reassurance thus: "the task while difficult, remains feasible" (Small *et al.* 2002: 203).

We argue that the task is no less simple and no more daunting than that of continuing to prop up the now vast, cumbersome and unworkable infra-structure many Anglophone countries have built around residual and forensic child protection services that are spending most of their time on controlling poor families rather than on identifying the cruel, the deviant, and the sexually predatory. Freymond and Cameron (2006) offer more reassurance and some sound advice on the matter of maintaining a new vision for child protection and safety. They suggest a range of possibilities for doing things differently, which include learning from the many countries and jurisdictions that have different philosophical starting points and that have gone down very different policy and practice paths in caring for children and families. In their outstand-ing contribution to the debate about how we develop positive systems of child and family welfare that work for different cultures and communities, they examine three generic historical approaches—family service, community care, and child protection. And they state in their conclusions:

> This book is an argument against continuing our insular discussions of child and family welfare, and an argument for opening ourselves to the possibilities of learning from others and to alternative ways of under-standing ... Our experiences with cross-national comparisons and dialogues, despite the substantial challenges involved, is that they are much needed tonics for imagining innovations and for renewing beliefs in the possibilities of building positive systems of child and family welfare.
>
> (Freymond and Cameron 2006: 316)

The history of child protection in recent times appears to be one increasingly dominated by technical–rational solutions involving surveillance of children and families; determining and measuring levels of risk; locating and punishing parents (particularly mothers); increasingly monitoring worker perform-ance; and relocating more and more troubled children to ever-decreasing numbers of foster homes and alternative care arrangements. Despite the lack of evidence of positive life and other outcomes of all of this, Anglophone countries seem to continue to keep tweaking the system to just do more of the same. In the next chapter, we suggest that re-examining and re-visioning the ethical and moral underpinnings of our work is an essential step in reforming our approach to child and family welfare systems and we provide a framework for how this might be done.

7 A new ethical and practice framework

There are clearly multiple competing interests and ideas implicit and explicit in this introduction to a chapter on ethics in child and family well-being practice. What principles can best guide practitioners who work in rule-governed environments, where one is at risk if one does not follow the rules? What do professional codes of ethics tell practitioners about how to manage in environments in which so many rights have to be balanced and so many rules and procedures followed? It has been difficult to find even a discussion about the ethical frameworks of child welfare practice in most of the now impressive tomes of child protection literature.

Most child protection manuals focus on policies and procedures, identify predictors of risk, and present risk assessment tools, propose a variety of checklists—and rarely mention ethics and values. An exception to this is the more recent handbook by editors Mallon and McCartt (2005) which notably deals with a variety of ethical tensions in child welfare practice. The primary policy framework in Anglophone countries has been a "rational-bureaucratic one of developing the law, procedures, audit, inspection and other forms of performance management" (Ferguson 2004: 206). The dominant principle that drives practice is "the best interests" of the child. How do professionals manage this internationally accepted imperative—to operationalize the "best interests of the child"—in environments dominated by fear, anxiety and proceduralism? How on earth does anyone, let alone a visiting professional or legal system, make any judgment about the "best interests" of the child that can actually predict a better short- or long-term outcome for the life of that child when our capacity for prediction is so patently poor? It is a truism to state that moral concern about risk to children and outrage about "bad" or "dangerous" parents and the failure of professionals to avert child death and injury has driven child protection practice rather than ethical debate about the nature of these interventions. Turnell and Edwards (1999) assert practice has been "problem saturated and risk dominated" and that we need to find another paradigm to inform our work (p. 181).

It is within this context, in which practitioners are understandably driven by the competing interests of concern for children, respect for families, fear for themselves as well as ever-demanding procedures and protocols, that we look to a value and ethical framework that might help with the disquiet that we and many practitioners and scholars feel. And, as has already been made evident in this book, child welfare and child protection practitioners are suffering from more than disquietude. There is a real poignancy in the sense of loneliness and isolation that practitioners articulate about the moral questions they struggle with—and so often they do this on their own (Holland and Kilpatrick 1991 cited in McAuliffe 2005: 1).

In his recent book, *Social Work in a Risk Society*, Webb (2006) makes the observation that in all its areas of practice—including child protection—social work is in danger of being consumed by risk-aversion and defensive practice, and is also in danger of losing its moral legitimacy. He suggests that, although now in need of revision, social work was based on a well-articulated ethical intent which, he argues, has become compromised if not lost in the highly individualistic and procedurally dominated practice domains of the late twentieth and early twenty-first centuries. He supports Kemshall's analysis that the role of social workers has shifted from meeting people's needs to a preoccupation with avoiding risk to themselves as well as others (Kemshall 2002). And he makes an urgent plea for social work to find a new ethically valid and functionally accountable model of practice, noting that "If risk society necessitates a life without guarantees, we require an ethical framework that acknowledges the continuity of care, recognition and strong values" (Webb 2006: 8).

One value explicitly used in much comment about child protection policy and practice that has permeated the literature and discourse over time is that of the primacy for the welfare of the child. And the one ethical principle that quite understandably appears to dominate, implicitly if not explicitly, is duty of care or the duty to protect the most vulnerable. More recently, and alongside of this, has emerged a focus on the rights of the child as articulated in the United Nations Convention on the Rights of the Child (UNCROC). Early in the history of child protection, the centrality of the rights of the family was articulated (NSPCC). And throughout its history, child protection practice has also continued to straddle the tension between the rights of children and the rights of parents. But these simple frames are now insufficient to help practitioners to address the complexity and intricacy of the decisions they face on a daily basis. The old paradigm was one in which we fought between the polar positions of the rights of the child and the rights of families—between a child focus and a family support focus (Parton 1991; Archard 1993; Fox Harding 1996; Berry 1997; Thomas 2002; Smith 2005).

Why is there such an absence of discussion about ethics compared to legal and procedural matters in the child protection literature? Does child protection practice really come down to competition between the rights of the child, the duty of professionals, and the rights of families? Or might the apparent lacunae in the debate mean that it is too hard to find an ethical framework that could be applied to such a contested area and across such a range of jurisdictions, disciplines and legislative arrangements and cultures? Might it mean that to propose any framework other than one that relies so heavily on the "best interests" principle, is to invite the chagrin of advocates that have fought long and hard, and largely succeeded, in highlighting the vulnerabilities and abuses of children, and thereby sees themselves and children at risk if the rights or needs of other stakeholders are addressed? It has been suggested that the risk that scholars and professionals face if they appeal to any framework other than a child rights one is to be accused of being too family (or mother) focused at the expense of the welfare of the child (Tronto 1993; Reich 2005). Here we aim to move beyond the misleading simplicity of a singular duty of care or child rights approach and acknowledge the complexity of the ethical decision making that is involved in maximizing children's well-being and safety.

What is ethics?

Very few people who work in child and family welfare have a background in philosophy, moral theory, or ethical reasoning, but most would have undertaken some lessons in ethics and ethical decision making during their professional education and training. For many, that learning occurred a long time ago. For some, there were no such lessons. And perhaps, for the majority, whatever they learned may bear little resemblance, and have little relevance, to what they experience in the world of child protection today. Following their research with practitioners about the basis of their moral reasoning, Asquith and Cheers (2001) confirmed the disquieting observation made by other scholars that "practitioners' personal moral frameworks are more frequently described as influential [in their decision making] rather than professional norms and codes of ethics" (p. 16). Of course, this would be fine if there were some assurances that personal frameworks were driven by other than idiosyncratic values.

Our suspicion is that for at least some workers, the only "ethical" framework they use is their personal sense of moral duty which they couple (perhaps with a greater or lesser degree of unease) with a regulatory framework that dictates procedures they have to follow (Oakley and Cocking 2001). And yet we have been aware that over the last couple of decades at least, there has been a growing awareness about ethical challenges in child protection (Clark 2000; Hugman 2005; Congress and McAuliffe 2006), an emerging alarm at the risks associated with poor decision making (Munro 1999b, 2002; Sinclair 2000; Pinkerton 2002; McConnell and Llewellyn 2005; Pecora *et al.* 2007), and a growing sense of concern about how to integrate proceduralism, values, and ethics (Meagher and Parton 2004; Gray and Gibbons 2007).

Some workers belong to professional associations that espouse a code of ethics. And, if they do, they would know that many such codes appear to capture ethics in terms of fairly simple values, principles such as respect, self-determination and justice (Banks 2006). Few, if any, of these codes provide a decision-making framework to assist the worker to utilize the code. As Banks (2006: 98) argues, this would not be possible and would be contradictory to the intention of such codes. When asked what they understand ethics to be, many human service workers respond by listing three principles—confidentiality, duty of care and self-determination.[1] In traditional Anglo-Saxon, individualistically framed professional codes developed by Anglophone professional associations, there is congruence around the common principles or features, and one would be forgiven for thinking that ethics is simple and static, and that all one has to do is simply apply moral principles to problems (Beckett and Maynard 2005; Banks 2006). It was clearly not the intention of the architects of such codes to give a misleading simplicity to their construction or to make them hard to apply consistently to practice situations. On the other hand, it is likely that these authors understood that moral and ethical reasoning have a long tradition and disciplinary history that to the newcomer may appear foreign, esoteric, and devoid of practical significance, and so their intention was to simplify the complex into meaningful elements.

Of course, ethical discourse is not static, nor is decision making simple. As Roger Smith so succinctly observes in his scholarly work about the place of values in the delivery of children's services:

> It is not possible ... to achieve successful interventions simply by following standardized lists or codes of practice. The help that these offer is limited in the context of challenging dilemmas or conflicting interests; it is at this point that professional skills and judgment must be applied.
>
> (Smith 2005: 8)

Ethical practice often requires us to make tough decisions in arenas that are fraught with difficulties, and in which emotions and conflict and ethical dilemmas abound. Although it might not appear obvious, the choice is generally not between what is clearly right or wrong but, rather, what is best or worst in the situation. Essentially, ethics is concerned with the morality of human behavior and can be described as the study of the standards by which we make decisions about the best things to do in circumstances in which we find ourselves (Darwall 2003).

Child protection is one of the most profoundly challenging and difficult areas of practice and it is clear that standards are increasingly contested. It is impossible to imagine how one could conduct one's business in child protection without confronting and appreciating the multitudes of moral questions that are a daily occurrence. Child protection practitioners cannot help but act in ways that will affect the lives of children, parents and communities—for a long time in to the future. They will have to make choices, individually or collectively, that will help or hurt people. In relation to this idea, Hinman

---

1 This observation is made by one of the authors who in presenting extensive ethics training with a range of professionals always asked the question about how participants understood the term ethics within their professional activity.

(2003) asserts: "we can ignore morality, but we cannot sidestep the choices to which morality is relevant" (p. 2). And, ultimately, social workers and other child protection practitioners, like all other professionals, have to review the fit between their moral and ethical sense and the "conventional demands of their role" (Oakley and Cocking 2001: 161).

In much of the material about the complexities of practice and decision making, and the tensions that have to be mediated by practitioners that have been identified so far, it would seem apparent that the ethical choices appear often to be stated in dyadic terms. That is, the choice is between the interests of the child and the interests of the parents; or, the choice is between principles such as duty of care and "best interest" or outcomes for children. Here, we take a view of ethics which sees it as being less about the principles alone, and certainly not about the rules and procedures alone, and more about how we incorporate those principles and procedures in order to work together to grow families and communities that flourish. Within this view, ethical practice is not about private morality and the acceptance of principles or procedural rules but, rather, it is about how we engage together in work that contributes to the development of a human and community "good." Furthermore, ethical practice is not just about *what* we do (the action)—it is about *how* we do it. And it is not just about what we do *with service users* but how we understand the societal mandate for what we do.

In presenting this framework we use the ideas of moral philosophers such as MacIntyre (1981) whose leading text *After Virtue*, and Thompson whose co-edited book, *Nursing Ethics* (Thompson *et al.* 2000) have provided much inspiration to our view that ethical practice is more than the application of ethical principles. As these moral philosophers argue, ethics is not just concerned with codes of ethics, or rules of behavior, or the consequences of actions, but is most importantly concerned with the means, context, and conditions for the flourishing of human societies. Within this approach to ethics, power sharing and avoidance of causing more harm than good are essential elements of a decision-making process and, to be more specific, practicing ethically involves sharing with others in problem-solving activities based on knowledge of principles and skills in their application.

For child protection and welfare practitioners, it is our view that practicing ethically must involve working with some important universal principles such as a duty of care to the vulnerable child but, as importantly, it involves working out how these principles are to be applied to intensely personal and private issues, while recognizing the rights of all stakeholders within a highly contentious, contested, and culturally diverse family and public environment. This approach to ethical practice requires that practitioners work in partnership with families and other stakeholders—an approach that requires considerable "practical wisdom," judgment and resilience because, in this framework, practitioners are professionals who own their professional judgment and cannot restrict themselves to procedural guidelines alone (Darwall 2003).

On the basis of their research and professional practice with families and research and training with workers, Turnell and Edwards (1999: 197) make a most relevant observation about this approach to ethics and professional practice that is seen to be respectful of the interests of a range of stakeholders and is not slavish to procedures. Their words remind us of Lipsky's (1980) observations about "street level bureaucrats" who, while operating in an environment fraught with uncertainty and resource shortage, do what they need to do by interpreting and implementing policy in ways that are contextually appropriate, rather than what protocols and policies dictate.

> Workers pursuing collaborative strategies often operate at the periphery of the protocols and conventions of normal agency practice because they feel that following the standard agency line is likely to alienate the client. Parents articulate the same dilemma in a more down-to-earth fashion when they receive services they perceive to be focused on protocol.
>
> (Turnell and Edwards 1999: 197)

Theoretical approaches to ethics

There are a number of ways of capturing the diverse history of ethics and moral theory and to engage with a formal summary of these in this short chapter would likely alienate most human service workers whose job is not moral theory but the practical pursuit of solutions to very real problems. A straightforward explanation we have found is one that is described well by Thompson *et al.* (2000), who distinguish between three primary ways of thinking about ethics.

Deontological (principalist) approaches

These are based on what are considered to be first principles, that is, the way to work out the right thing to do is to resort to obligatory moral positions such as "always tell the truth." Some deontologists would argue that all ethical decision making is determined by a set of rules which define our duties and rights. Doing our duty might mean in this context "always giving priority to the rights of the child," or "always acting in the best interests of the child." Ethical decision making here simply means trying to answer the question, "what rules should I follow?" From this point of view the consequences of an action are irrelevant to whether it is the right/wrong thing to do: the judgment about what to do is solely dependent on following the rules/principles. In this case, even if the outcome is "bad," poor ethical judgment cannot be blamed because the rules were followed.

Teleological (consequentialist) approaches

This ethical approach focuses on outcomes, that is, one strives to achieve the best thing in the circumstances, by choosing to do what the person believes will produce the best outcome. Decisions are made on the basis of what actions will produce the most benefit to individuals (act utilitarianism), what actions will cause the least pain, or what policy will result in the greatest good for the greatest number (rule utilitarianism). In these cases the way to work out the "right" thing to do or the right policy is to work out which is likely to have the most beneficial consequences. A teleological position is not necessarily synonymous with pragmatism. The decisions here are based on the question, "what sort of long-term ends should I pursue?," rather than "what is the most practical solution?"

From this point of view it is not clear by what criteria we are to assess costs and benefits of actions or policies. And it is certainly not clear how such an approach in child protection practice might measure outcomes. It is interesting to note that the "best interest principle," while appearing at first glance to be captured in a deontological or principalist approach, contains an implicit assumption about consequences or outcomes. That is, one would expect that it would need to require an answer to the question "what is in the long-term interests of the child?" It is also interesting to note that a teleological approach could assist practitioners to engage with an analysis of "what is in the long-term interests of the child as well as the family and the community?"

Hogdkin and Newell (1998) maintain that the principle of the "best interest of the child" forms the core principle in child welfare and dominates practice internationally. If this is the guiding principle, what does it mean to workers and how is it to be explained to parents and families? What behaviors does it demand? It appears to be a principle but in reality, it assumes a known outcome. It directs actions and decisions toward an unspecified end point where supposedly the interests of the child will be clearly realized. If it is an outcome, what means or predictions are used to justify it? How valid are such predictions unless they incorporate a long-term view of the vagaries of a child's development into an adult? What practitioners tell us is that the best interest is often measured by what is relevant in the "here and now." Herein, contemporary issues and risk assessments predominate, rather than any longer-term perspective.

Virtue ethics

Virtue ethics emphasizes the cultivation of the virtues, or the moral character of the decision maker, as a necessary condition for sound ethical decision making (McBeath and Webb 2002). One description of virtue as used by Aristotle is that of the habit of being able to choose the mean between extremes. Aristotle suggested that this capacity for discernment requires a depth of character and a capacity for prudence rather than an articulation of rules. Virtue ethics stands in contrast to the two other approaches which emphasize either the duty to obey rules, or to make consequences of actions the touchstone of one's morality and decision making. In virtue ethics competent decisions are based on a mixture of knowledge and skilled judgment or practical wisdom (McBeath and Webb 2002). This must be informed by real experience, and not just abstract principles or anticipation of future consequences.

What virtue ethics emphasizes is that the quality of the decision and action is mediated by the integrity, practical wisdom and competence of the decision maker (in this instance, the child protection practitioner). If one follows a virtue ethics approach one acknowledges that what the child protection practitioner needs to do in order to apply principles "correctly" is to have the ability to understand the context, articulate the important elements within it, and to anticipate possible outcomes (MacIntyre 1981; McBeath and Webb 2002). What scholars of moral theory encourage us to do is to revisit the foundational work of philosophers such as Aristotle who argued that good decision making and personal integrity are linked to "character" and to "practical wisdom." This means that the best decisions are made when people have acquired moral competence, which is based on excellence in judgment and the ability to integrate knowledge and experience. They assert that good decisions cannot be made by simply, or blindly, or even bureaucratically, applying a set of rules and procedures.

A deontologist may point to the fact that they will be acting in accordance with a moral rule such as "do unto others as you would have them do unto you"; a teleologist may argue that they hope the consequences of doing something will maximize well-being; and a virtue ethicist may argue that helping someone is a good or benevolent act in its own right. The philosopher Niebuhr (1963) argues that our actions are not so easily categorized, that is, they are neither simply rule-governed, nor simply aimed at achieving idealistic goals, but are a bit of both—they are aimed at acting responsibly and responsively in relationships of tension. Tobin (1994), a contemporary writer about virtue ethics, captures the nexus between approaches and the subsequent complexity thus: "Ethics is about doing the right thing and—more importantly—about being the kind of person who can be relied upon to do the right thing" (Tobin 1994: 55).

In a virtue ethics framework, the practitioner provides the bridge between principles and outcomes—"what virtue ethics emphasizes is that the quality of the action produced is affected by the integrity and competence of the moral agent" (Thompson *et al.* 2000: 303). There has been a significant development in recent years in conceptualizing ethics for professional practice (Hugman 2005; Banks 2006; Weber 2006) and a particular growth in interest in the "ethic of care" (Meagher and Parton 2004), which some authors see as a form of virtue ethics. The latter approach to ethics for practice in the caring professions dates from the seminal work of Gilligan (1982) and, as developed by Tronto (1993), and then expanded by writers such as Webb (2006), places the reciprocal caring relationship at the center of all human endeavor and, it is suggested, offers a very useful framework to assist child and family well-being practitioners to move beyond simplistic principle-based approaches to the care and protection of children.

Ethical practice for child and family well-being

Arguably, the understanding of ethics by many child protection practitioners continues to be dominated by models learned in early education or teaching about professional codes of ethics or codes of conduct and, arguably, the way principles are uncritically presented within these codes or rule books. Undoubtedly, their thinking is also dominated by the burgeoning procedures, protocols, and risk assessment tools described elsewhere—procedures that are developed and reified as mechanisms that, if followed, will supposedly safeguard the welfare of children and ensure best outcomes for the child.

By reintroducing virtue ethics to the repertoire of understanding about ethics we are making the point that action-guiding rules cannot be applied reliably or correctly without practical wisdom, because correct application requires situational appreciation of the contextualities. That is, child and family well-being practitioners—whether they have the formal title of child protection worker or not—need to develop the capacity to recognize, in any particular situation, those features of it that are morally salient, and those people whose welfare will be affected by any decision they take. For them, sound ethical practice is about contextualized decision making rather than policies that dictate a "one size fits all" approach (Barton and Welbourne 2005). But it does beg the question about how, in the sorts of risk-averse, media-sensitive, and punitive child protection environments in which people work, does one assist practitioners to develop practical wisdom and competence rather than simply follow rules (or even standard procedures and tools) in their decision making?

Professional codes of ethics can only give practitioners a range of core ethical principles to guide practice and help them manage their decision making. Most current legislation and departmental policies include large sections on core principles that should underpin decision making. Yet, the descriptions of the practice environment provided throughout this book give some insight into the limitations of this approach and support the case for a more "realistic" approach to decision making that takes account of the complexity of the processes involved, and the difficult situations that child welfare practitioners have to address.

In our view, much contemporary child protection decision making is fundamentally flawed by its focus on managing immediate risks and risk avoidance, as the fundamental imperatives. These are rhetorically justified by appeal to "the best interests of the child" and tend to be based on ignorance of longer-term impacts on the well-being of children and their location within their families and communities.

The managerial context for ethical practice

We have already referred to, and much has been written about, the fact that professionals working with children and families in adversity, while aiming to protect children from significant harm, are working in environments that are increasingly risk-focused, ambiguous, demanding and demoralizing (Howe 1992; Lawrence 2004; Parton 2006a). Working in neoliberal political environments where NPM abounds—with limited resources at their disposal, and where demands for economic constraint, reduced taxes and government expenditure drive social policy—child protection practitioners have to deal with some of the most marginalized and disadvantaged people in our communities. Practitioners are being asked to safeguard children and balance the rights of families and communities at the same time as having to cope with a sensationalist media ever ready to point an accusing finger at them or at the families they meet (who are seen to have failed as parents). In these circumstances, professional accountability is often akin to public retribution and blaming.

It is also apparent that many workers are not ethically trained or equipped with the skills to deal with the new organizational priorities and mechanisms within which they have to work (Lonne *et al.* 2004). Perhaps it is not surprising that it is a worldwide phenomenon that front-line workers in child welfare are increasingly hard to recruit, resign quickly and burn out at a rapid rate (Stanley and Goddard 2002; Stevens and Higgins 2002; Bednar 2003; Littlechild 2005).

Rabbi Neuberger (2005), offers a powerful critique of the way we manage vulnerability in our society, and questions whether the present care system works to anyone's benefit. She argues strongly for a return to "a different [respectful] attitude toward social workers" (p. 191) and front-line workers:

> At present we have a risk averse society, more concerned with stopping one child murder—however awful—than with supporting dozens if not hundreds of vulnerable youngsters via a system that places full trust in the judgement of professionals.
>
> (Neuberger 2005: 126)

If Neuberger and others are right, and our communities and press have lost faith in the judgment of child welfare workers, then it is necessary if their judgment is to be trusted again, that professionals are able to articulate the moral principles on which their judgments are made (deontological), subject these to rigorous scrutiny in terms of their assessed outcomes (teleological), and embrace the challenges of being present as competent moral agents who don't simply follow procedures but apply these with prudence (virtue). It might seem perverse to state this, but professionals need to feel safe in order to secure the safety of children and families. They need to be protected from the threat of becoming victims of moral panics themselves (Jenkins 1998), of being objects of punitive criticism in a culture of blame (MacDonald 1990; Reder *et al.* 1993) or being seen to be driven by the risk-aversive policies of politicians (Parton *et al.* 1997; Kemshall 2002).

In the contemporary neoliberal managerial environment which is preoccupied with procedures, rationing and rules, there is an urgent need to reawaken the values necessary for the enlightened ethical practice that Neuberger describes. Practitioners exist in an environment that generates fear and defensiveness and promotes ever greater reliance on procedures, regulations and a narrow pursuit of professional survival. It is in this risk-averse neoliberal environment, and within the current conditions of "profound uncertainty," that Webb (2006) asserts "we need to take steps to reawaken core ethical practices and activate the moral sources of social work" (p. 233).

Theoretical framework

In revisiting the ethical foundations of child welfare practice it is imperative to adopt a new ethical stance. There are three conceptual elements which, we argue, form the crux of a new framework for ethical decision making that will promote child and family and community well-being. These elements will, we argue, enable us to start to meet the challenges named by researchers, commentators, and scholars, reported by practitioners, and echoed by young people and families who are caught up in the web of child welfare practice today. We have called these three conceptual elements: *competing ethical principles*, *unequal power relationships*, and *complex stakeholder responsibilities*.

Competing ethical principles

The three competing ethical principles that are central to all decision making, and are always in tension in any given society, are beneficence, justice and respect for persons (Thompson *et al.* 2000). These principles feature in some of the earliest known codes of ethics and law, and have served as a foundation for the development of modern biomedical and social ethics (Beauchamp and Childress 2001). Beneficence (often referred to as the duty of care) constitutes the duty to do good rather than harm, to protect the weak, and to defend the rights of those who can't defend their own. Justice represents the duty to treat people as ends in themselves and never as means to an end, to be fair and equitable to all, and to avoid discrimination. Respect for persons contains the duty to value the rights, autonomy and dignity of all people and in so doing to be truthful and honest with them, because in doing otherwise, one is not respecting them.

Contained within the principle of respect for persons is the duty of confidentiality, that is, if we value others we respect their right to privacy (Thompson *et al.* 2000). Given that confidentiality is a fraught issue in all human services let alone in child protection practice, understanding this derivation of confidentiality is, to our minds, more useful than conceptualizing it only in the simple legalistic way so often adopted by policy makers and practitioners. This idea is not new and Clark's (2000) observations in relation to confidentiality are valuable in helping us to realize the importance of finding a new ethical direction: "the whole concept of confidentiality appears inadequately defined and decidedly threadbare in practice" and "the traditional principle of confidentiality is based on a mistake of means for ends" (p. 189). Confidentiality is a precept that is unquestionably located in every disciplinary code. We argue that it is a dangerously deceptive expectation and must be re-conceptualized as an outcome of an analysis of the place of various principles (particularly but not only that of respect) and applied to all stakeholders—aptly called "moral subjects" by Clark—who are involved in a situation requiring decision making

The principle of "duty of care" sits most easily with an understanding of childhood and vulnerability. No sensible person would suggest that adults don't have a duty to care for and protect children. We have already identified that in the current risk-averse and managerially dominated environment, the prime activity associated with the duty of care to children relates to the assessments or predictions of risk and likelihood of harm. This carries the accompanying duty to protect any child from harm. In reality this is often a highly speculative endeavor where, unless great attention is paid to the context and relationships, imponderables and subjective values determine our understanding of duty and drive us to impute certainty to our knowledge of outcomes. Prediction of risk is, by every definition, a most inexact science! Yet it has won almost universal favor as the guiding criterion for determining duty of care for children and for allocating resources. As Kemshall (2002) indicates, "risk" has replaced "need" as a determinant of the duty to provide a service.

Justice and respect for persons are two principles that can, and must, be held in tension with the duty of care, in all ethical decision-making processes, and certainly when one is considering the well-being of children. Yet, we argue, these other principles are often overlooked as the preoccupation of statutory workers and the legal advisory system coalesce and potentially collude around "the best interests of the child." Barbara Hudson (2003) argues that "justice is under threat in the risk society" (p. 203). Those who are seen to be the source of the risk are considered less worthy and they become of themselves, "bad," "less worthy," or "dangerous." Child protection literature is replete with such terms and labels. And, in considering risks to children, in our risk-averse society the individuals who are held primarily responsible are the natural parents. Indeed, as Urek (2005) and others argue, it is the "bad mother" who is primarily named and shamed. A preoccupation with the procedures of risk assessment threatens to ignore issues of justice (non-discrimination) and it also threatens the duty we have in a moral community to respect or value the humanity and dignity of all other stakeholders (rather than just the child). In this instance, the main threat to the integrity of the ethical decision-making process is that of excluding the fundamental respect that is owed to parents: human beings who are themselves in trouble (Sennett 2003).

Power

All relationships mediate power. Indeed, ethics is about power in relation-ships and the basis of power-sharing within them (Thompson *et al.* 2000).

Professionals working in child protection typically work with people who have little power (Thorpe 1994; Dale 2004), and yet practitioners are in situations where they have access to much power themselves. When parents meet with professionals they confront formal statutory power (people employed by the state to carry out its duties), coercive power (people who can take their children away), and expert power (people who are expected to have a scientific knowledge base). It is unsurprising that, in his recent research with parents, Dumbrill found that "the way parents perceive workers using power was shown to be the primary influence shaping their views and responses to child protection intervention" (Dumbrill 2006: 27).

By and large, people who are reported for abusing and neglecting their children come from communities with little structural power. They are generally poor, from Indigenous or culturally and linguistically diverse communities, are single parents, or have a mental health, intellectual, addiction, or other health problem (Melton and Thompson 2002; Spratt and Callan 2004). And their access to financial, legal or personal resources is severely constrained. McConnell and Llewellyn (2005) state this concern forcefully: "children removed by child protection authorities typically come from poor and marginalized families" but "the cruel and uncaring parent mythologized in the media is rarely encountered in child protection practice" (p. 554). Indeed, one has to wonder whether the widespread demonizing of abusive and neglecting parents has been carried out with the political purpose of justifying the significant powers given to child protection authorities on behalf of the state.

McConnell and Llewellyn (2005) argue that in not recognizing their own power and the inherent powerlessness of these families, professional practitioners are subscribing to the depoliticization of social inequality. There is, of course, the counter argument to this that the child is even more vulnerable than either of the relatively powerless parents or carers and that it is our duty to protect the most powerless person—the child (Tew 2006). Within this latter argument there sits the assumption that there is a need for a forced "either/ or" choice rather than a need to acknowledge the fluidity of power and the indeterminacy of power differentials between various stakeholders. In his very recent publication, Tew presents an excellent multidimensional matrix of power (protective, cooperative, oppressive or collusive) that he says enables workers to pay attention to the different ways that they can use the power they have, and helps them to acknowledge the relative powerlessness of the various service users they meet. For the purposes of this book, Tew's (2006) is a timely construction of power, for in his words, it is one "that does not have an inherent tendency to put down the service user and define them as someone who is essentially inadequate, needy or dangerous" (p. 48).

Complex stakeholder relationships

Ethical decision making in child and family well-being, like all decision making, demands a process in which competing duties to various stakeholders need to be factored into the analysis without jeopardizing the practitioner's primary duty to a vulnerable child. Yet, in conceptualizing ethical decision making in child welfare, one could be forgiven for believing that, as Scott and O'Neil (1996) have critically observed, child protection practice tends to simply apply the principle of duty of care in the dyadic relationship between abused children and the professionals who rescue them. In this model, the child is seen as being in need of protection by the worker (who has a duty to protect him/her). Where a child has been intentionally and seriously harmed by an adult, no one would deny that there is an immediate and absolute duty to remove and protect that child. However, while there has been a longstanding emphasis on the importance of family when a child's welfare concerns are being mediated, it is only more recently that the complexity of these and other stakeholder relationships have become pronounced in child protection decision making. These stakeholders have been referred to by some as the "unheard clients" (Dale 2004; Kapp and Vella 2004).

It is evident that there are indeed multiple stakeholders involved in most child and family well-being decisions. Clearly, the first stakeholder is the child whose well-being and safety are paramount and the second is the parent who, while being reported for harming or failing to provide appropriate care for their child, is still a human being deserving of respect. It is impossible to understand the work of child protection professionals without taking account of the ethical duties workers have to another stakeholder—their employing authority. Fourth, the public and the media are stakeholders and there are significant pressures to conform to media expectations of child protection. Next, child and family well-being practitioners cannot ignore the views of those adults who have experienced child protection investigations or the care system (Australian Senate Community Affairs References Committee 2005). These stakeholders represent a community who have much legitimacy to comment on the successes and failures of the child welfare system—and many of them tell profoundly disturbing stories about the failure of the "best interests of the child principle." Finally, it is increasingly clear that the other stakeholders in this journey, siblings, foster parents and grandparents, also expect and require respect, and for their concerns and needs to be heard. As a consequence, all professionals working in child and family well-being need to become aware that they may be required to conceptualize and articulate the decision-making task more comprehensively, and to recognize its complexity.

It is our argument that this requirement for acknowledging complexity has always been present, although a preoccupation with procedures and the acceptance of simplistic deontological approaches have tended to obscure the significance of multiple stakeholder interests in assessing and ensuring child safety. Additionally, we emphasize that child and family well-being practitioners have a responsibility to apply the three ethical principles of beneficence, justice and respect for persons to all major stakeholders involved in the lives of each child—recognizing that decisions have to be made about what priority is given to which principle in each case. It is not sufficient to say that one only has a duty of care to a vulnerable child.

What is the duty of the child and family well-being practitioner to the parent of the vulnerable child? Sadly, much recent research informs us of what we know anecdotally and that is that few parents experience respect in relation to child protection practice (Freymond 2003; Dale 2004; Holland and Scourfield 2004; Thomson and Thorpe 2004; Freymond and Cameron 2006). It would be hard to find a morally acceptable argument that practitioners dismiss the needs of the biological parents of that child—as if the relationship of the child to the parents is incidental to the welfare of the child. Furthermore, in our virtues framework for child protection practice, decision-making processes must embrace a critical analysis of the contextual variables present in each specific case. These variables include poverty and illness, not so much as indicators of risk, but more as needs and as potential avenues for assistance. Finally, any assessment of the risk of harm should specifically include an examination of the longer-term outcomes as well as the immediate and pressing issues of safety.

Implications for child and family well-being practice

There is a vast amount of evidence which tells us that those who are investigating child protection complaints are primarily investigating children and families who are marginalized by factors such as: illness, poverty, disability, single parenthood, and ethnic minority status (Thorpe 1994; McConnell and Llewellyn 2005). Yet the dominant child protection assessment model is one focused on determining whether a parent (generally the mother) is suitable (Sinclair 2000; Urek 2005) and whether a child or children are "at risk" from parents (generally the mother). Contemporary child protection practice will remain bedevilled by the demonstrable shortcomings of a predominantly linear and limited deontological ethical decision-making framework, which fails to take into account the context of power relations and their complexity unless it engages with the alternative approaches encompassed herein. Child and family well-being practice must face the challenge to develop a strong value base in which a duty to protect children is balanced with the principle of respect for all people involved, and where the principle of justice is permitted to find a place back at the decision-making table.

With the new organizational imperatives associated with increasing risk aversion in public life and public policy, and media alarmism, both creating increased pressures to interventionist policies in child welfare practice (Parton 2006a), there is an even more urgent need to make value-based judgments that care for children in an atmosphere of genuine respect and partnership with families and communities. It is important to rebuild trust in the decision-making competence of child and family well-being practitioners.

Professionals in child and family well-being have a tough job making decisions about the welfare of children that recognize the vagaries of real life, under conditions of uncertainty, where they have limited resources, face overwhelming proceduralization and confront the relentless risk of judgment by management and media. Reframing ethical decision making in child welfare within a virtue ethics framework offers us a critically important opportunity to deal with these factors more realistically and compassionately and that recognizes their complexity and the centrality of the practitioner in judgment making. Virtue-based and prudential ethical decision making requires child and family well-being practitioners to consider and balance different principles, respect the rights of multiple stakeholders, understand the demands of the specific context, face the uncertainty of judgments about immediate and longer-term outcomes, and face the challenge to become professionals of integrity who not only do the right thing but are the sort of people who do the right thing.

As Sennett (2003) argues so powerfully in his thesis on the ethical duty of respect for persons, we must re-engage with the justice imperative that "in society, and particularly in the post-welfare state, the nub of the problem we face is how the strong practise respect towards those destined to remain weak" (p. 263). Respect the particular vulnerability of children we must, but the potentially weak are not only the children, they are very likely to be the families and communities who belong to these children—people who are, by and large, those who experience what some have called "unearned disadvantage"—an issue dealt with so very well by Waldfogel (1998) and others.

The challenge for policy makers and practitioners is as substantial as it is significant for future generations of children, families and communities. How do we turn around a juggernaut that is fueled by the powerful imagery of defenceless children but, more poignantly, lubricated by media images of "statistically rare" children who have suffered terrible injuries at the hands of more powerful people in whose care they were entrusted? The organizational systems that we have developed to protect children have been incrementally built on the foundations of what are seen to be child protection failures (Stanley and Manthorpe 2004). The death of any child is unpalatable. But what are the iatrogenic consequences of developing organizational systems that are expected to do the impossible—protect every child from harm?

Child protection practitioners generally work in an unenviable "dilemmatic space" (Bauman 1993), in which uncertainty and risk intensify anxiety and where any attempt at the reflection that is required for the ethical decision making outlined above is likely to be sabotaged by the fear of failure and shame (Froggett 2002; Watson and Moran 2005). In these situations, a retreat to rule books of protocols and procedures is the seductive and only safe solution for weary and wary workers unless we restructure organizations to facilitate value-based conscious reflective practice and judgment. Scholars such as Waldfogel (1998) and others saw the need for dramatic change to child welfare practices to be urgent over a decade ago. Indeed, Hessle presents the ongoing urgency more recently and most provocatively in a language which is hard hitting. In reflecting on the failures of the past and planning for a future he urges us to end "the costly experimentation with children by child welfare" (Hessle 2000: 4). In the next chapter we consider the importance of organizational shifts that will enable the different kind of work that is now required of child and family well-being practice if we are to realize any hope of the change that is needed—a change that is guided by a strong ethical framework that values continuity of culture, community, and family as quintessentially central to the life of every child.

There are considerable difficulties experienced in practicing in respectful and just ways in contemporary child protection structures and organizations where NPM dominates and power is used overtly and covertly to control staff and service users alike. We argue that to re-establish needed and beneficial helping and working relationships as the norm, and thereby successfully implement a new ethical and practice framework, there also has to be reform of the organizational structures and service delivery model to make them more effective in addressing the needs of children and families and improving their safety and well-being. Nevertheless, irrespective of agreement or otherwise with our proposed structures or indeed the current ones, the principles and ethical framework we have outlined have to be embraced in order to prevent child abuse and neglect and render much needed help to those caught up in these destructive behaviors.

8 Effective organizational and service delivery models

Informal social care responses to address and prevent child abuse and neglect occur daily in a myriad of ways including a grandparent caring for their grandchildren, neighbors lending a hand by providing food and nurturing, and a friend assisting with support and aid to help a distressed parent. On the other hand, *formal social care* responses are delivered by the community through organizations and, in the case of child protection systems, we examined their chronic failings in Chapter 4. In this chapter we outline how the many problems that currently exist in these policy making and service delivery mechanisms can be attended to, and in many instances, satisfactorily addressed. We do not claim that our suggested frameworks are ideal—every organizational system has its own strengths and problems. However, they will probably make substantial improvements upon the current structural and organizational approaches to the vexed issues entailed in preventing child abuse and neglect.

We recognize that structural reorganizations have a history of solving some problems while creating new ones. We are also mindful that the process of reforming child protection will take time. Nunno (2006) suggests that changing dysfunctional organizational cultures takes 5–7 years, and the sort of systemic change that we propose will also take time to plan, implement and then bed down so that helping rather than punitive cultures can thrive (Smith and Donovan 2003).

Importantly, we also recognize that there are no panaceas to the current state of affairs. We do not offer an "off the shelf" model that can be easily transferred to every community location. As we have seen with evidence-based practice, it is critical that knowledge be contextualized to a particular social and community situation if it is to be effective (McDonald *et al.* 2003; Whiting Blome and Steib 2004; Barton and Welbourne 2005). Essentially, service delivery models and programs must be contextually appropriate and address the unique requirements of a particular social and cultural milieu, community and child protection system. For example, the transfer of a forensic US system into rural and regional Vietnamese communities is likely to be unsuccessful as the local infrastructure, customs, and values are quite different (P. Meemaduma personal communication April 26, 2007). We are not suggesting that the proposed models are appropriate for every set of community and organizational circumstances, or that they should be forcefully imposed on contextually incongruent situations. Fitting square pegs into round holes is self-defeating.

Rather, we put forward key principles and themes that, in combination with the suggested structures, can be adapted to local circumstances and contexts. What specific structural arrangements and form agencies and services should take needs to be matched to the local political, cultural, and organizational contexts, keeping in mind the principles and themes we put forward. We also acknowledge the inherent difficulties and limitations of terminology when advocating for major reforms across a variety of community contexts, where the same term can mean quite different things for people in diverse situations and in different historical times. The most obvious example is the term child protection itself, which tends to range from the most specific of targeted services to a broader inclusion of what many would see as much of family support and more generalized child welfare services. With these limitations and caveats acknowledged, we hope that our proposals will help to facilitate critical and creative thinking to address the identified system problems and serve the community better than at present.

The core problems to be addressed

Earlier on we identified a broad range of issues and failings in contemporary child protection systems. The complexity of these problems and their inter-connectedness make it difficult to know where to start the task of reform. To assist this process we have identified what we believe are the core problems that need attention. For ease of understanding we have separated these into two categories, those that are primarily but not exclusively related to: structural arrangements; and, practice processes and mechanisms. It is acknowledged that, among other things, structural-, ideological-, and practice-related influences shape these problems and their manifestations within child protection systems (Ferguson 2004; Merrick 2006).

Issues related to structural arrangements

- The societal mission provided to contemporary child protection organizations has become far too broad and diffuse, leaving managers and practitioners with impossibly incongruent goals and objectives.
- Current approaches to the provision of social care are overtly punitive, with the child protection system geared for the surveillance and control of specific groups in the community, such as the poor, single women, Indigenous people, and those with disabilities. Moreover, it has become a system where, generally speaking, help is neither available nor accessible, with many parents either fearing the system, or unable to engage with it, particularly men (Scourfield 2003, 2006).

- The child protection system is oriented toward ceasing rather than restoring relationships, with retributive justice approaches dominating.
- Forensic interventions are deficits-oriented, and strengths-based perspectives tend to be in tension with the value and practice framework of child protection (Smith and Donovan 2003; Holland and Scourfield 2004).
- There is an over-focusing on tertiary rather than primary and secondary prevention (Shireman 2003), with programs being poorly integrated with broader economic and social welfare systems of government and society.
- Generally speaking, organizational cultures are deeply dysfunctional, being characterized as crisis-driven, power-laden and coercive, abusive, closed, and defensive.
- NPM approaches are oriented toward political rather than practice considerations, with executives and managers often unable to effectively relate to the complex, contested and conflicted nature of child welfare work. Moreover, notwithstanding NPM's self-promoting claims of superior performance, there is little research to demonstrate best approaches to management in these systems (Wells 2006).
- Child protection organizations, despite rhetoric such as "partnership" and "community," are typically large bureaucracies that are separated from, rather than embedded within, the neighborhoods and communities they are supposed to serve.
- Alternative care systems are broadly failing, being overburdened and increasingly incapable of meeting the reasonable demands made on them by the community, parents and children (Pecora *et al.* 2003, 2005; Shireman 2003; Courtney and Dworsky 2006; Stein 2006). Too often they are temporary and unsafe. The needs of children in care, by definition those with the highest needs and risk, are largely at the forgotten end of the child protection process. Nevertheless, large-scale placement breakdown is a primary contributor to the crisis-culture that drives much of child protection practice. While there is a large systemic emphasis on accountability, in reality, there is little by way of real support, treatment, therapy, and monitoring on offer.
- Indigenous peoples are grossly over-represented in child protection systems around the globe, with the present-day structural and community issues of poor health, economic, and social indicators being directly related to significant historical events including colonization and systemic racism (Johnston 1983; Cunneen and Libesman 2000; Shireman 2003).

Issues related to practice processes and mechanisms

- Over time, definitions of child abuse and neglect embraced notions of "harm" and "risk," and expanded to be all encompassing. They now have little discriminatory ability to screen out the ordinary vicissitudes of family life and relationships, effectively reframing all parental–child relationships as harmful. This definitional imprecision, in combination with other structural and organizational factors, has contributed to the blow-out in reports and workload focused on risk of harm rather than demonstrated need (Shireman 2003; Mansell 2006a,b; D. Scott 2006a).

- Despite being the key platform in which child protection services are delivered, there is compelling empirical and anecdotal evidence of widespread failures existing in the working relationships between staff and service users, particularly parents and men (Scourfield 2003, 2006). Relationships are not so much characterized by trust, empathy, caring, and respect, but distrust, judgmental attitudes, conflict, and misuse of power. That these problems occur with professional practitioners who are trained to "use themselves" as facilitators of change is quite disturbing.

- Generally speaking, there is a lack of a clearly articulated value and ethical base in practice frameworks, with reliance upon technical tools and proceduralized policies to determine the nature of service delivery and practice (Froggett 2002). This has worked to the clear disadvantage of children, parents, and families who are usually poorly informed about the "rules of engagement" and left to their own devices to determine appropriate standards of professional practice.

- While case management has considerable benefits, particularly from a management perspective, it lacks focus on the criticality of relationship and nature of personal change, and generally applies a short-term change time frame that is unrealistic and largely unachievable by most parents (Froggett 2002).

While other problems are apparent, addressing these matters will go a long way toward developing a system that is humane, caring and able to provide the sorts of services required by children and families in need, including increased safety and support.

Principles and themes for reform

Building on our earlier values and ethical framework, it is important to describe the sorts of themes and principles that should characterize a reformed child protection system. Without a genuinely value-derived and driven approach to practice, a community's social care programs are without a clear moral basis, "the heart," necessary for interventions into the private lives of its citizens. Programs need a value base lest they primarily become instruments of social control and oppression. What is evident is that within contemporary society, social care programs must not only have a moral basis, but also be justifiable on economic and social grounds. We agree with Eric Scott's (2006) and Bill Jordan's (2006, 2007) arguments that a focus on child and family well-being is a suitable conceptual and practical framework for reforming child protection and achieving a just, humane and self-sustaining society.

The values and ethics outlined in Chapter 8 have to be integrated throughout a reformed child protection and welfare system. They are inseparable ingredients from sound, ethical and just governance, policy and practice. Hence, they are both implicit and explicit in the organizational and service delivery models we propose. In addition, there are number of key principles and themes that should underpin and guide reformation of the organizational, programatic and practice domains. However, as noted earlier, these categorizations are not clearly delineated within the realities of contemporary social systems. For example, the principle of a renewed emphasis upon local neighborhood/community and prevention is located in the program domain, but it is also important in the organizational and practice domains. Separating where these three levels begin and end is not as important as understanding that the principles may apply primarily with one, but still be relevant to the others. With this in mind, the following outline of relevant themes and principles for a reformed system are offered.

The organizational domain

The organizational domain entails: Accessible and available services; Utilizing a public health model that accepts programatic risk; Adoption of a "safety" culture by child and family well-being organizations; Appointing practice-informed management; Embracing accountable and responsible management; Employing well supported, guided and managed staff; and, Developing organizational capacity for the issues affecting Indigenous peoples to be addressed.

The organizational domain is a critical area in need of reform as current structures are failing. For services to be truly effective in meeting the needs of children and families, they need to be easily accessible and available, that is, based locally and open at the hours that are needed by them. Moreover, the services should embrace strengths-based practice approaches rather than deficits-oriented ones.

Dorothy Scott (2006a,b) has mounted a convincing argument for utilizing a public health service-delivery model for child welfare services. Among other things, this entails broad acceptance of programatic risk with cases of abuse and neglect measured per 100,000 children, and identifies that keeping every child safe from harm is impossible.

Adoption of a "safety" culture by child and family well-being organizations is required to improve communications and reduce the risks of serious events, such as preventable child deaths and serious injuries. Safety cultures are used by organizations where there is a small risk of an incident that will have significant adverse repercussions (e.g. airlines), and are based on a shared behavior of effective and timely communication of critical information to those who need it in order to prevent catastrophic events (Westrum 2004). Within fragmented and overwhelmed child protection systems, such a culture entails an explicit acceptance of the imperfect communication and coordination that exists, with protocols and practitioner responsibility needed to expedite critical information.

Child and family well-being organizations need managers who are practice-informed and can embrace the need for practice values, knowledge and skills at all organizational levels. A significant shortcoming of NPM is that its discourse does not resonate well with professional practitioners, whose narratives tend to be centered on the issues and efficacy of helping interventions (CMC 2004). Hence, an altered management discourse is required that relates to, incorporates, and values the professional discourse.

Truly accountable and responsible management and service delivery to vulnerable people requires a significant shift away from narrow NPM notions of performance and quality (Tilbury 2004, 2006). Rather, its focus is on developing, measuring and monitoring performance indicators that accurately reflect the real impacts and outcomes upon the well-being of children and families. Practice-related and client-focused evaluation is required. Moreover, broad organizational and systemic performance indicators need to be used so that the real outcomes for the well-being of families and children are examined, rather than merely those matters that are in agency interests (Tilbury 2006). For example, we need to examine accountability in governance, agency, and program links to community, and the ability of particular programs and services to meet identified priority needs, as well as undertaking broader research on systemic and client outcomes, organizational cultures, and climates.

Effective child welfare organizations depend upon a well supported, guided, and managed staff. For management teams to be successful in changing counterproductive cultures and practices, trust is required between the various staff groups. By attending to staff needs for social and emotional support, ensuring that quality professional supervision, development and training is accessible, and providing adequate role and practice direction, management can genuinely engage with staff about the need for altered behaviors and approaches as part of a reform agenda.

The effects of institutional racism and colonization have been devastating to Indigenous peoples around the world, with their communities, families, and cultures subject to longstanding destruction, through practices such as child removal and adoption (Johnston 1983; Cunneen and Libesman 2000; Hill 2000; Neu and Therrien 2003; Zapf 2004). Furthermore, Indigenous children continue to be grossly disproportionate within contemporary child protection and alternative care systems (Shireman 2003). Dominant child protection and child saving ideologies have been largely unable to incorporate Indigenous cultural practices and beliefs into their operations, although many good initiatives have been tried (Hill 2000). There is a critical need to develop the systemic and organizational capacity of Indigenous peoples and organizations if these problems are to be successfully addressed.

The program domain

The principles and themes for the program domain center on the need to realign the approach to child abuse and neglect from a punitive and blaming orientation toward one that fosters choice by children and families, and genuine partnerships that facilitate support, assistance and treatment. The program domain themes and principles include: Rebalancing social care and social control mandates; Promoting service user choice rather than coercion; Embracing restorative justice approaches; Establishing "confidential places" where family members can access help without fear of mandatory reporting; A renewed emphasis on local neighborhood/community and prevention; and Reducing reports and false positives/negatives (Munro 2002).

Child protection programs need fundamental realignment of their under-pinning ideologies and resultant practices in order to rebalance the social care and social control functions. While statutory programs undertake neces-sary social control of child abuse and neglect, this needs to occur within a clear legal framework that provides protection for the vulnerable, as well as accountability and rights for all parties. The legal system principles to ensure these occur in a balanced, responsible and measured way should be as clearly articulated as they are in the criminal justice system (Pelton 2008).

Child and family well-being systems need to embrace the principle of parental and children's choice rather than coercion, except in those situations where there is an immediate threat of serious child abuse and neglect occur-ring. If we are to encourage people to seek assistance to prevent abuse and neglect we must reward their efforts rather than punish them.

Programs must embrace the principles and approaches of restorative justice in order to attend to the damaged relationships that child abuse and neglect can cause (Braithwaite 2004; Burford and Adams 2004). Processes and forums for negotiation and mediation of the complex issues at hand need to be intertwined within programs and at all stages of intervention (Turnell and Edwards 1999; Adams and Chandler 2004; Crampton 2004; Holland and Scourfield 2004; Pennell 2004). This necessitates a sharing of power between children, parents, families and child protection practitioners, who retain statu-tory authority to intervene when necessary and appropriate to protect children from serious child abuse and neglect (Neff 2004; Dumbrill 2006). Promotion of reflective practices by staff is a necessity for changing problematic organizational cultures and promoting altered relationships with service users (Froggett 2002; Fook 2004).

There is a critical need for "confidential spaces" within these systems for children and parents to seek therapeutic assistance without the explicit threat of statutory intervention, thereby putting preventative treatment ahead of punitive retribution. These sorts of programs are successful in a number of locations including Belgium (Cooper *et al.* 2003; Freymond and Cameron 2006) and in Western Australia's SafeCare confidential program that provides support, counseling, and treatment services to families where child sexual abuse is an issue (C. Chamarette personal communication November 24, 2006). While these approaches run counter to the predominant mandatory reporting approach, they offer a capacity for openness and disclosure that, with appropriate safeguards in place, can help families to restore relationships, protect the vulnerable, and prevent further abuse. Such approaches directly meet the needs of many abused and neglected children who just want the abuse to stop and their familial relationships to remain intact. Current approaches largely ignore their plea.

An emphasis on programs being embedded within, and relating directly to citizens in, local neighborhoods and communities is in dire need of renewal (Melton and Thompson 2002; Jack 2004; Hornberger and Briar-Lawson 2005). Generally speaking, as child protection systems have grown into large proceduralized bureaucracies, they have become increasingly focused on internal issues rather than on linking with local community stakeholders and citizens. This has decreased the emphasis on primary and secondary prevention programs being developed and delivered locally, preference instead being given to national and regional prevention programs.

Child welfare programs should aim to reduce the negative impacts of investigation false positives and negatives. Trawling through copious volumes of unproven allegations and reports wastes resources and diverts attention from those cases that are serious and warrant statutory intervention to protect vulnerable children (Munro 1999b; Ainsworth and Hanson 2006), and overwhelms systems (Shireman 2003; Mansell 2006a,b; D. Scott 2006a). Moreover, current programs give scant attention to the social and other costs of intrusive investigation of innocent people. Ultimately these well-intentioned invasions of privacy bring child protection systems into a cycle of negative public perception that is counterproductive to their reliance upon public information to uncover and respond to abuse and neglect.

The practice domain

It needs to be acknowledged that some child protection advocates can be reluctant to embrace further reform because of their high degree of personal commitment to the needs of abused and neglected children (Melton and Thompson 2002; Nunno 2006), which can lead them to see a change in direction as a lessening of the societal obligation to protect them (Mildred 2003). Second, many practitioners are change-fatigued from the almost endless organizational restructurings, and policy and procedural alterations. Nevertheless, in our view, most practitioners realize that the present way of protecting children is not working, and is probably unworkable and unsustainable. Without practitioners embracing the reforms we outline here, there is little chance of positive change (Nunno 2006). The key principles and themes in this domain are: Emphasizing the criticality of relationship-based practice; Emphasizing the long-term and holistic focus to care and assistance; Reflective practice; and Promoting worker discretion and creativity.

Recently there has been increasing attention paid to the criticality of relationship as a medium for change in social welfare generally, and in child protection in particular (Turnell and Edwards 1999; Froggett 2002; Smith and Donovan 2003; Ruch 2005; de Boer and Coady 2007). We see these calls as evidence of the failure of many policies, programs and practices that are underpinned by neoliberal ideologies, a deficit-orientation, over-reliance on punishment as a behavioral motivator, and the elevation of individualism over communal responses. Children who are abused and neglected and those who harm them are typically in turmoil and pain, desperate to find an alternative way of functioning, and seeking succour and nurturing from the social care systems set up to address this. Without establishing empathic, caring, and compassionate relationships, effective treatment and therapy is impossible, and personal change and development unlikely. Staff utilization of reflective practice in their relationships should be the foundation and core business of child welfare and well-being. Reflective practice by staff regarding their relationships with service users is essential if child protection systems are to change this fundamental aspect of protective and helping interventions (Froggett 2002; Fook 2004).

Practice interventions need to be long term and holistically oriented in providing care and assistance to needy children, parents, and carers. Staff need to have the requisite knowledge, skills, and program support to provide this. Case management systems have tended to adopt short-term and narrowly targeted practice in order to keep interventions within policy and eligibility guidelines and under budget. This is short-sighted and completely at variance with those needing services due to issues of abuse and neglect, who typically have longstanding, multiple, and complex social and personal problems that cannot be simply "fixed overnight." Indeed, setting short-term interventions as the guide often sets these people up with an impossible deadline for change—"set up to fail."

Without increased worker autonomy and discretion to intervene creatively then practice will remain deadened by hollow and unproductive procedures that are largely unhelpful to those in need (Froggett 2002; Cooper *et al.* 2003; Gupta and Blewett 2007). Sadly, the necessary artistic elements involved in social care and therapeutic practice have become dominated by an over-reliance upon technically oriented evidence-based practice (EBP), misapplied to inappropriate contexts. This said, practitioners should not be "laws unto themselves" and there needs to be appropriate levels of responsibility taken and accountability measures in place.

Structural rearrangements and realignments

There are many structural factors affecting the incidence of child abuse, and in particular neglect, which is typically the largest category of harm experienced by children (Shireman 2003). Issues such as poor housing, unemployment, poverty, low educational achievement, racism, poor health and mental health, and disability play critical parts in the processes that lead people to have contact with child protection authorities (Melton and Thompson 2002; Shireman 2003; Spratt and Callan 2004). However, the system response is often more likely to be a hindrance to them rather than a help, with assistance tending to not be provided even though protective issues are identified (Shireman 2003; Pelton 2008). A whole-of-community response is required to address these sorts of systemic issues, but government plays a key role in both the provision of statutory interventions necessary to attend to serious child abuse and neglect and, where necessary, to remove children from dangerous situations, as well as the coordination and integration of holistic responses that address the underlying causes.

However, the current missions given to child protection organizations are too broad, hotly contested among diverse stakeholders and, hence, unachievable. The diverse and unclear nature of the mission and subsequent functions renders them prone to chronic failure through repeated poor performance in combination with political persistence to see them carry on their roles. We offer a viable alternative to this by making the organizational missions clear and achievable, with separate functions for different agencies, within an integrated comprehensive system of service provision. We recognized that this is "easier said than done" (Merrick 2006: 213). Nevertheless, along with others, we view the combination of roles such as protection to all children, investigation, surveillance, prevention and early intervention, assistance and support to families, provision of alternative care placements, and guardianship of children in care as seemingly impossible for any single agency to handle (Parton 1997; Cooper *et al.* 2003; Pelton 2008). Moreover, these sometimes competing and incongruent roles and associated functions are immensely confusing to those people who come into contact with child protection organizations. While trust in organizations has largely replaced trust in individual helping professionals, the chronic failure of child protection agencies has left many children, parents, and carers with nowhere to place their trust (Munro 2004a; Butler and Drakeford 2005). We believe that altered structural arrangements are an important step in facilitating the rebuilding of service user trust in the capacity of the child and family well-being system to help people in need and to protect the vulnerable.

The avalanche of child protection reports and investigations, even with differential response, have overwhelmed child protection agencies (Shireman 2003, D. Scott 2006a) and rendered them incapable of meeting their missions, and prone to unacceptable levels of false positives and false negatives (Mansell 2006a,b). We argue that to rectify this, legislative and policy change is urgently needed to redefine and narrow the current basis for legal interventions. A narrower definition and interpretation will alter the current risk-aversive "catch all" definitions that show no concern for the damage caused by unsubstantiated examinations on people's lives or the subsequent harm to an already overloaded and failing system (D. Scott 2006a). Intrusive investigations would be reduced, enabling greater social care responses to address children's and families' needs. Importantly, these changes necessarily shift attention and resources away from forensic investigation and assessment to early intervention and preventative services (Waldfogel 1998, 2008). They enable a far more beneficial and less coercive provision of assistance and support to children and families to be available, thereby enhancing their well-being in tangible ways. In essence, social care and social control are rebalanced with increased opportunities for service user choices. Services are more likely to be provided on a "needs," rather than a "risk," basis.

In our view there are four discrete primary functions which are probably best given to different agencies to carry out, namely:

A   Child protection—a court-based agency having responsibility for the investigation of allegations of serious abuse and neglect including criminal offences against children, and any resultant legal action to protect children such as assessment, removal, and continuation of existing protective court orders.
B   Child and family well-being programs—a statutory organization providing social care to assist and support children who are not under court orders, parents and families with a range of needs, and where the standard of care is of concern but is not able to be classified as involving serious abuse and neglect.
C   Services for children under court orders and their families—a statutory organization implementing all court orders relating to the guardianship and care of children and their families, including alternative care arrangements, treatment and therapeutic interventions, and reunifications.
D   Human service agencies providing community-based assistance and support—these include all the existing non-government, faith-based, not-for-profit and for-profit agencies and practitioners who deliver social care programs and services to children, parents, and carers. They do this on either a free or fee-paying basis, or alternatively under contract or other arrangement to agencies A, B, and C above, being accessed voluntarily by children and families in need.

Agency A—Child protection

There will always be a need for an organization to undertake a child protection function, including intrusive investigations and other statutory interventions because, sadly, some people can be dangerous to children and their well-being, even if unintentionally. Vulnerable children need to be protected from acts which may cause them significant harm. Agency A's organizational mission could be to receive, investigate and assess reports of serious child abuse and neglect and criminal offences against children and, where appropriate, reach a negotiated outcome with the parties concerned to ensure the safety of the child but, if necessary, put the matter before a court to determine the merits of a protective order. Our view is that this necessary function should be limited to those cases where statutory interventions are clearly necessary and warranted. This can best be achieved within an integrated public health model that also focuses on prevention programs that aim to reduce the rate of child abuse and neglect per 100,000 children, rather than a system that adopts counter-productive risk-averse approaches while attempting to prevent all harm to children (D. Scott 2006a,b; Testro and Peltola 2007).

There should also be clearly defined checks and balances to these sorts of coercive powers and authority. In many, but not all, Western nations the key accountability is to a court or a tribunal, often a special Children's Court jurisdiction. However, in those countries that have an adversarial judicial system, significant tensions and conflicts can arise between the parties and personalities (Ashford 2006; Freymond and Cameron 2006). In some European countries the tradition is for the court to be an inquisitorial process where the judge has the role of independently investigating the circumstances at hand, determining the facts at issue and dispensing justice accordingly (Freymond and Cameron 2006). We believe that there is considerable merit in the child protection function being the direct responsibility of an independent inquisitorial Children's and Families Court, which could be staffed by judges and independent investigators including lawyers, police officers, social workers and human service practitioners. There are examples around the world where specialist investigatory teams of this sort operate successfully (Freymond and Cameron 2006; Pelton 2008). To establish cultural congruency and address over-representation issues it is critical to have Indigenous staff members in those communities where Indigenous children are entering the child protection system (Hill 2000; Freymond and Cameron 2006). This is particularly the case in rural/remote and urban communities that identify as Indigenous.

Agency A would probably be better placed near a hospital in order to provide around-the-clock access to specialist medical and other allied health personnel (Cooper *et al.* 2003). Staff would make appropriate enquiries to establish the facts at issue when allegations of suspected serious abuse and criminal offences against children are received. In circumstances where the matter did not warrant further intrusive investigation or court involvement, the child and family could be referred to Agencies B, C, and D, depending on the precise need and circumstances. The adoption of a system-wide "safety culture" is essential for the rapid flow of information that indicates children are vulnerable to serious abuse and neglect or criminal offences (Westrum 2004). Many child death inquiries have identified that agencies and personnel were aware that children were at significant risk but did not pass on critical information (Munro 2004b). A "safety culture" goes some way toward addressing this problem.

When a child's immediate safety or a serious long-term consequence requires protective orders, court-appointed investigators could apply for them. A judge of the Children's and Families Court could make orders when satisfied that the existing civil burden of proof, on the balance of probabilities, was met and that a protective order was necessary. The independent Children's and Families Court staff could be authorized to apply to the court for protective and related orders (e.g. for medical/psycho-social assessments, orders for the removal of an offender from the household). Assessments and other services might be accessed through any of Agencies B, C, and D on an inter-agency agreement or contract basis. Criminal prosecution would remain within existing criminal jurisdictions, using the current standard of proof for criminal matters.

Importantly, an inquisitorial jurisdiction gathers the facts and seeks to find the best outcomes for the children concerned, rather than being focused on establishing the guilt or otherwise of a parent or carer. When child abuse and neglect occur there is nearly always damage to the child–parent or carer relationship. Hence, the Children's and Families Court would favor utilizing restorative justice principles and approaches to directly attend to the conflicts and other issues between the family members, with negotiation and mediation used to find and explore possible solutions. There is growing support for the positive impact of a range of restorative justice approaches such as Family Group Conferences (Cooper *et al.* 2003; Burford and Adams 2004; Holland and Scourfield 2004; Neff 2004; Pennell 2004; Pelton 2008), particularly for Indigenous peoples (Freymond and Cameron 2006). A forensic approach to child protection does not necessarily have to taint the relationships with parents, particularly where there is a strong policy and practice emphasis on working collaboratively with service users, treating people with respect and using power appropriately (Turnell and Edwards 1999; Cooper *et al.* 2003; Dale 2004; Holland and Scourfield 2004; Dumbrill 2006). Within a court setting, parents are more likely to see the processes and personnel as fair and objective (Ashford 2006), a critical element in their acceptance of interventions. However, these approaches are compatible with a strengths-based and constructive assessment process (Turnell and Edwards 1999; Parton and O'Byrne 2000; Holland and Scourfield 2004). Nevertheless, these approaches are not a panacea and there is a small percentage of adults who will be difficult or impossible to work with no matter how good the processes and practitioners (Hill *et al.* 2002).

A number of measures are needed for child protection organizations to be congruent with, and embedded within, their local neighborhood/community contexts, and for there to be a coordinated agenda for addressing child and family well-being (Melton and Thompson 2002; Cooper *et al.* 2003; Jack 2004; Hornberger and Briar-Lawson 2005; Freymond and Cameron 2006). For example, in Queensland Australia, the Crime and Misconduct Commission (2004) recommended that there be senior Child Safety Directors appointed to all major government departments as part of the reform of the child protection system in Queensland, Australia. This innovation has been reasonably successful in elevating child protection onto whole-of-government agendas and provides an effective mechanism for coordination and implementation of change across organizations. In our proposed system, Child and Family

Well-being Directors could take on these inter-organizational and system coordination roles. Further, the Children's and Families Court might have nominees appointed to the local Community Child and Family Well-being Boards that are established to over-see the child well-being system processes and outcomes, and provide feedback and guidance about how best to implement programs and deliver services. We will explore this later in greater detail.

In our view, a separate investigatory body within a specialist court structure with inquisitor authority and processes is well placed to address the critical issues. First, the social mandate and mission for this organization is clear—to investigate reports of serious child abuse and neglect and, when warranted, to initiate protective action. Second, it allows the rule and due process of law to be applied to the decision making about specific protective intrusions into the private lives of citizens. Third, it places a much needed brake on the demand processes leading to spiralling reports and overloaded systems (Shireman 2003; Mansell 2006a,b) by having a strong legislative regime for setting the benchmarks for intrusive measures. Fourth, it clearly separates the social control from the social care roles, which can provide greater role clarity for children, parents, carers, and social care practitioners. Fifth, while providing protective interventions, the use of restorative justice forums and a strengths-based orientation makes it more likely to find satisfactory negotiated solutions in statutory interventions. Sixth, locations near hospitals make access and availability much easier for service users. Finally, it enables committed and specially qualified and trained staff to undertake the necessary intrusive investigatory role within a process that is answerable and accountable to a court.

Agency B—Child and family well-being programs

Current child protection systems largely fail to provide any meaningful and accessible help to those in need, even when protective interventions are warranted (Shireman 2003; Pelton 2008). In our proposed structure, strong emphasis is placed upon providing integrated primary, secondary, and tertiary prevention and early intervention services to children, parents and carers who are in need. This is delivered within an integrated public health model (D. Scott 2006b), with Agency B primarily responsible for direct service delivery of child and family well-being programs and referral to funded neighborhood/ community-based agencies and service providers (Agencies C and D).

Having separate organizations doing investigations and providing assistance and support seems important for rebalancing the social control and social care functions. These around-the-clock services must be easily accessible and available because families often experience crises outside regular business hours. A combination for this agency of hospital-, neighborhood-, and community-based locations (such as schools and shopping centers) will likely achieve this, with the former being open all hours for emergencies as well as appointments. Staffing should be multidisciplinary, including nurses and allied health therapists, with access to hospital medical specialists. Indigenous staff are necessary in communities where Indigenous children are over-represented (Johnston 1983; Hill 2000). Having available professional help and treatment, practical support and assistance will help turn around the current child protection system from one which often blames, punishes, and hinders attempts by people to get aid, to one which renders tangible assistance in non-judgmental strengths-building ways.

Critically, Agency B needs sufficient resources to realize its clear and achievable mission—To provide a range of accessible, high-quality prevention and treatment programs and services to children and families in need, with priority given to those likely to come into contact with the child protection system. A primary orientation toward helping enables citizens to meet their needs, with improved child and family well-being the achievable outcomes. Hence, the organization must be an integrated one that balances early intervention and prevention, and tertiary prevention. Moreover, while the organization might be the main point of access and referral for initial assessments and assistance, it could also have primary responsibility for planning, coordinating, and funding the range of programs and services delivered by Agencies C and D. A central role seems likely in the provision of social care to children and families, with priority to those who are subject to protective and guardianship orders.

Agency B could have a key role in providing voluntary preventative visiting services to families in need for issues such as parenting skills and assistance, practical aid and help, behavior management, treatment and therapy for past abuse and neglect, and general support services. Referrals or court orders for assessment and assistance could be received from the Children's and Families Court and Agency C, for those children and families requiring specialized services to prevent them entering further into the statutory system or who are already subject to a protective order—a recognized high priority group that is often unable to access help. This integrated system would facilitate reciprocal referral arrangements between organizations.

Adopting a strict case management approach to service delivery in Agency B seems likely to fail children, families, and carers, because it fundamentally alters their relationship with practitioners into a "managing" function rather than a helping one (Froggett 2002). Furthermore, case management functions appear as part of the complex equation leading to decreased staff autonomy and discretion, and increased job dissatisfaction and turnover, because they fail to adequately address practitioners' helping motivations. While casework has its limitations, it is not beyond realignment into a robust practice process that focuses on the primacy of the relationship for providing help, and also meets the legitimate management requirements for oversight, documentation, accountability, and prioritization. To be fully effective in these extremely complex and difficult helping relationships with children and parents, practitioners need to have organizational latitude for discretionary decision making and innovation (Glisson and Hemmelgarn 1998; Turnell and Edwards 1999; Froggett 2002; Cooper *et al.* 2003; Freymond and Cameron 2006). Overt and controlling risk-averse and accountability (blaming) messages from management are likely to shut down the very capacity for innovative therapeutic relationships that many service users want and need. Stunted and sterile proceduralized approaches are a death knell to facilitating the sorts of changes in children, parents, and carers that are required to prevent abuse and neglect.

Our integrated child and family well-being systems need strong linkages between all agencies, but also between other government agencies that have responsibility for areas that are structural influences upon child and family well-being, such as income support, education, housing, health, mental health, police, etc. Appointing Child and Family Well-being Directors in senior government posts can help to achieve this, along with Agency B taking the lead agency role in promoting child and family well-being.

Agency B organizational units need to be connected and embedded within the community so that their policies and practices remain grounded in the realities and values of local citizens (Melton and Thompson 2002; Cooper *et al.* 2003; Jack 2004; Hornberger and Briar-Lawson 2005), particularly in Indigenous communities (Johnston 1983; Freymond and Cameron 2006). One way to achieve this is to establish local Community Child and Family Well-being Boards, perhaps with Agency B chairing these structures, which could have key roles in over-seeing system processes and outcomes, and providing feedback and guidance about policies and service delivery. The involvement of a range of community stakeholders, service users, and luminaries can provide an important mechanism for ensuring that the organizational culture is open about its methods and accountable to those who come into contact with it—characteristics which contemporary child protection systems do not always share (Cooper *et al.* 2003). For genuine reform to occur, it is critical for both service users and Indigenous community members to have a voice that is heard within these forums (Froggett 2002). The role of service users in mental health reforms provides a good example of how productive service user input can be to service development.

Importantly, Agency B differs from many child protection organizations because a "safety culture" is embraced as a key principle for its operations and communication, emphasizing staff responsibility to ensure that information is passed on to those who "need to know" in order to protect the immediate safety of children and protect them from serious harm, as well as to facilitate service user access to programs and services. Without this culture and its associated practices, the primary orientation of Agency B toward helping seems unbalanced and unable to properly protect children. Nevertheless, it remains impossible to guarantee that any system can achieve even near-perfect communication transfer. A public health model recognizes and accepts these limitations.

An important caveat is that within Agency B there needs to be "confidential spaces" (Cooper *et al.* 2003) for parents and children to be able to freely disclose without the undue fear that doing so will result in blaming and punitive responses from the agency. The significant drawbacks to helping children and families from mandatory reporting are increasingly evident (Harries and Clare 2002; Blaskett and Taylor 2003; Melton 2005; Pelton 2008). "Confidential spaces" (Cooper *et al.* 2003) seem crucial forums for providing help for those who have been involved in abuse and neglect events but just want it to stop, and receive treatment, rather than an accusatory and punitive response from authorities. Agencies such as SafeCare in Western Australia (SafeCare 2007) have strict policies that allow confidential disclosures within a regime of ongoing intensive treatment and close monitoring to ensure children are safe from further abuse. The right balance can be struck in such programs between disclosure of abuse and the prevention of further incidents, without a "one size fits all" mandatory reporting and punishment approach.

Agency C—Services for children under court orders and their families

The third element to our proposed structural realignment entails a separate organization that is responsible for all children (and their families) who are subject to temporary and longer term protective court orders. This might include guardianship and care of children in alternative care placements, as well as treatment and therapeutic interventions for them and their families, and facilitation of reunifications. These children and their families have high needs, evidenced by a court determination that statutory intervention was warranted. Yet, in most contemporary child protection systems we find that insufficient resources are directed to address their needs, often because forensic investigations are getting priority. There is compelling evidence that the outcomes for children in care are generally unsatisfactory (Pecora *et al.* 2003, 2005; Shireman 2003; Courtney and Dworsky 2006; Osborn and Delfabbro 2006; Stein 2006; Berridge 2007) and that the state has largely failed in its "loco parentis" duties and obligations, moral and otherwise.

A single organization that has an unambiguously targeted group seems best placed to address their complex needs with a clear mission: To provide high quality assistance and services to children under protective court orders and their families in order to prevent further episodes of serious child abuse and neglect, and thereby significantly enhance their quality of life, family relationships, and life outcomes. To achieve this, Agency C might require:

- legislative authority and resources to enforce and implement court orders;
- an ethos of being a "model parent" to children in care including promoting and monitoring their safety and development;
- robust therapy and treatment capability for children and their families; and
- wherever possible and appropriate to actively work toward, perhaps using restorative justice approaches, reunification of the family, and if this is

not possible to ensure that any contact is to the short- and long-term benefit of the child.

Agency C would require substantial funding to purchase necessary treatments, therapy and other assistance from Agency B and Agency D community-based sources as required. Approaches that recognize the criticality of intensive, multimodal assessments and interventions immediately court action is taken are best to ensure opportunities for successful therapy and change are seized. However, a narrow case management system that "manages" families and has unrealistic time frames for parents and others to address their significant problems seems counterproductive, and we therefore advocate a therapeutic casework approach which emphasizes relationship as the starting point for successful change processes.

Because families who have entered the statutory system often experience a range of strong, volatile and mixed emotions, we believe that Agency C needs to embrace the restorative justice approaches and mediation/negotiation forums outlined earlier. The special nature of the "loco parentis" and guardianship relationship requires staff at Agency C to have a child-centered orientation that is based on the knowledge that the overwhelming majority of children are best served by ending the abuse and neglect, preventing repeat incidents, addressing the effects of harm on their social, physical, emotional and psychological well-being, and facilitating their lifelong relationships with their parents and families.

Agency C needs to be integrated and communicative with other parts of the system if it is to be effective and efficient. Inter-agency forums are essential if the overall system is to provide real help to those in need. While coordination is important, we nevertheless acknowledge that uncoordinated systems have also been found to offer families a great range of alternative access points for services (Glisson and Hemmelgarn 1998). Court-ordered and over-seen case coordination and decision-making mechanisms within Agency C are important as they offer independent case review and can be quite effective in making sure that children and families have a right of appeal of their case-related decisions. Because Agency C works with children and families at the serious end of the spectrum there is a need for clear communication flow to make sure that children are not exposed to unacceptable risks of serious injury and harm. Therefore, in accordance with a "safety culture" there needs to be clear protocols with other agencies, particularly Agency A, to ensure that information is provided promptly to those in a position to act in a protective way.

Because of the high needs and vulnerabilities of children in care, there needs to be a number of external accountability mechanisms in place. Establishing overarching and local Community Child and Family Well-being Boards seems one way of achieving this. Enabling community, service user and Indigenous representatives to have input into policy making and organizational directions is likely to ensure that programs and services are contextually appropriate and relevant to local neighborhood/community needs and priorities (Froggett 2002; Melton and Thompson 2002; Jack 2004; Hornberger and Briar-Lawson 2005). Other monitoring and accountability measures are also required for children who are in alternative care placements and an external court-appointed Guardians *ad litem* system appears more likely to result in an individual having a consistent longer-term relationship and contact with the child than is currently possible within alternative care and fostering systems, where numerous placements are typical (Osborn and Delfabbro 2006; Stein 2006). Moreover, it encourages an independent committed person to over-see the work of Agency C.

D Group Agencies—Providing community-based support and assistance

The protection and well-being of children is everybody's business (whole-of-society) and we advocate a robust role for non-government organization (NGO) and community-based family support agencies. The benefits that flow to families and children from having good access to neighborhood/community-based programs and services that provide needed help are self evident. They operate with a diverse range of organizational missions, but share stated objectives of providing social care to those in need, typically in a partnership with families. While having a broad range of services increases the likelihood of a lack of coordination, the benefits for families in need of acquiring available assistance are worth it (Glisson and Hemmelgarn 1998). The existing non-government, faith-based, not-for-profit and for-profit agencies and practitioners who deliver social care programs and services to children, parents, and carers are a vital source of help and a key prevention measure. These agencies and practitioners provide a web of social care and illustrate that children's safety and well-being are a whole-of-community and whole-of-society responsibility. Without their substantial contributions, the statutory-based agencies that we propose might be overwhelmed and unable to operate effectively (Shireman 2003) and there is less service user choice available.

Indigenous people require services and programs that are embedded within their culture and are attuned to their world views. Taken overall, there is a long and tragic history of the failure of mainstream agencies to provide effective assistance and to protect vulnerable Indigenous children and families, people who are subject to significantly worse economic, social, and health disadvantage than the rest of the community (Johnston 1983; Cunneen and Libesman 2000; Freymond and Cameron 2006). In view of the history of colonization, child welfare abuses and scandals, and cultural destruction through practices such as denial of language and familial/community connection, Indigenous people are understandably wary of mainstream programs. This is not to suggest that Indigenous run agencies are a panacea or that they are problem-free. Rather, that tangible expressions of self-determination and culturally congruent service delivery are important to all cultures, and more so for Indigenous communities due to the history of destructive contact with child welfare policy and practice. Local Indigenous community control of well-resourced social care services and agencies is necessary to ensure that the significant disadvantage is turned around.

All agencies and their services need to be appropriately resourced if early intervention and prevention is to be promoted, particularly because they attract clients on a voluntary partnership basis. It is our belief that the funds redirected from those unnecessary, counterproductive and intrusive investigations of families will go a fair way, but not all the distance, in meeting Agency D resource needs. These agencies operate on either a free or fee-paying basis, but could also work through contractual and other arrangements to Agencies A, B and C. Diverse funding sources make it more likely that the range of family and community needs can be responsively addressed, and that they are more able to operate with independence and flexibility. As key stakeholders, their involvement in Community Child and Family Well-being Boards would be beneficial. Because of the emphasis on voluntary service delivery, D group agencies are vital linkages between a revitalized child and family well-being system and the community.

Our proposed structure is not a "one size fits all" model for every neighborhood/community context. Rather, we offer it as one coherent and integrated way to address the problems that are apparent within most, but not all, child protection systems. To be effective in providing social care and social control measures that address the complex factors that lead to child abuse and neglect, these structures and processes need to be contextualized to the specific social and community situations they are located in (McDonald *et al.* 2003; Smith and Donovan 2003; Whiting Blome and Steib 2004; Barton and Welbourne 2005). Service delivery models and programs need to be adapted so that they properly respond to the unique social and cultural milieu and the needs of local children, families, and carers. Importantly, they reorient existing child protection system values and approaches to be more attuned to providing real assistance in a preventative way, rather than blaming, punishing, and ostracizing parents, and abandoning children to an alternative care system that is clearly unable, in system terms, to provide them with satisfactory help and positive life outcomes. However, to move from an existing dysfunctional child protection system to the new structures and processes outlined here requires detailed planning and change management processes, and it is to this that we now turn our attention.

9 Planning and implementing change

In this chapter we overview prior attempts at reform and change management in child protection systems and explore why these have often been unsuccessful and, in some cases, counterproductive. We will then outline our principles and themes for guiding the change processes, followed by proposals for effecting reforms at the broad societal and organizational levels. A central tenet of these processes must be the engagement of the broad community in the provision of social care, and decision making and planning about how to most effectively prevent child abuse and neglect within a modern civil society that adheres to notions of ethical practice, fairness, and justice.

We concur with Melton's (2005: 16) claim that the "Zeitgeist is changing" in child protection. This bodes well for the advent of the proposed reforms, which are likely to be well received by those who have an interest in promoting the well-being of children and families. In this chapter we outline the principles, processes, and measures to bring these reforms to a reality. To undertake the scale of reforms that we advocate will require a "dialogue of consensus" (Hirsch and De Soucey 2006: 172) that embraces systemic and organizational restructuring as being positive and necessary steps to improve and develop the social care responses to children and families in need, and to enhance their well-being. Moreover, this needs to occur within social institutions and organizations that have experienced almost continual change to their social mandates, missions, structures, processes and practices, often in politically driven circumstances. The end result has sometimes been change fatigue among staff who have to undertake transformations to the ways in which they think and work. Despite this, we remain convinced that most frontline and managerial staff will welcome and champion the ethical and practice framework we have put forward.

We are under no illusions about the size and scope of the reforms we have put forward. Taken together, they involve profound changes to the ways in which the safety and well-being of children and families are conceptualized, prioritized, and achieved. Ours is an ambitious program that involves a fundamental rethink and reshaping of the relationships between children, parents, and the state (Cooper *et al.* 2003). Structural, legislative, policy, and practice changes are involved, all of which require the support and imprimatur of government, which has critical responsibilities in this regard.

As noted in the *Scottish Executive Child Protection Review* (Hill *et al.* 2002), it is possible to transfer ideas like the ones we have suggested across nations and systems, but care must be taken to ensure they are contextually appropriate to the local situation and circumstances (Barton and Welbourne 2005). Similarly, there are many different approaches that can be taken to ensure the sorts of change processes take place to bring about the proposed system reforms. Hence, we are not suggesting that an uncritical or slavish application of our suggestions will be appropriate in every neighborhood, community, and nation. Rather, with child protection systems different in each community, albeit with many common elements and variations around central themes and approaches, contextualized change processes need to be congruent with local needs and issues. Furthermore, changing organizational structures and cultures does not usually happen quickly and can take 5–7 years of commitment and hard work (Nunno 2006), especially if there is significant resistance from key stakeholders (Westrum 2004). Change may need to be quicker or slower depending on local and organizational contexts. To implement our proposed changes, a number of important and influential factors need to be taken into account, including:

•   the broad cultural beliefs, priorities, and discourses about children and families etc;
•   the ideological underpinnings and the broad community mandate;
•   the amount, type, and nature of formal/informal social care systems;
•   the mission/s given to child protection and child welfare agencies;
•   the current degree of forensic approach adopted within these agencies; and
•   the capacity of local communities to be engaged and involved in change processes that affect them.

There is a variety of stakeholders, agendas, and priorities regarding children's welfare, and different groups have particular interests, viewpoints, and positions in relation to child abuse and neglect, and the efficacy of child protection systems and other related issues. For example, the recent study in the USA of prominent child sexual abuse "claims makers" found that the positions taken reflected moral, political, and scientific issues and that the most acrimonious differences centered on disagreements about the credibility of claims (Mildred 2003). Nevertheless, there is a significant amount of general consensus in relation to the need for societal interventions to prevent child abuse and neglect. In our view, there is also a growing realization among a range of child advocates that the current system is failing and is in urgent need of rethinking and reform (Cooper *et al.* 2003; Shireman 2003; Melton 2005; Freymond and Cameron 2006; D. Scott 2006a; Testro and Peltola 2007; Pelton 2008). Moreover, a majority view is that there needs to be an effective system for preventing abuse, including a state-sanctioned intervention into family life balanced with the provision of assistance to those struggling families subject to immense pressure within rapidly changing economic and social systems. This is particularly the case for groups over-represented in child protection systems. We posit that notwithstanding areas of significant difference, there remains a broad and strong social mandate for the prevention of child abuse and neglect, and hence for an effective system for achieving this.

Failed changed management

Change management processes are needed to reform child protection systems, but the historical record of previous efforts have been very mixed and, at times, counterproductive. That there have been many concerted attempts around the globe to reform child protection systems is beyond question. These have often followed the release of adverse findings from judicial inquiries into child deaths and other scandals, such as organized "abuse rings" (Hill 1990; CMC 2004; Munro 2004b; Parton 2006a). Changes have typically involved the recon-figuration of structural arrangements and responsibilities, new legislation and policy directions concerning who should receive interventions and services (e.g. introduction of differential responses), and the introduction of new procedures and ICT. These developments have aimed at achieving outcomes such as instituting more rigorous and consistent investigation and assess-ment procedures, preventing tragic child deaths, improving inter-agency coordination, and limiting professional discretion and increasing external accountability, particularly for children in alternative care (Hill 1990; Munro 2004b; Lonne and Thomson 2005). Of particular concern to the success of progress in child protection has been the propensity of judicially based inquiries and child death reviews to advocate for a host of legalistic, bureaucratic and procedural changes which have sometimes added to the problems within child protection agencies (Munro 2004a,b; Connolly and Doolan 2006, 2007). Unfortunately, this has often resulted in increased managerialization and practitioners becoming further detached from a helping role (Aronson and Sammon 2000; Jones 2001; Cooper *et al.* 2003; Smith and Donovan 2003; Parton 2007), which is often their primary motivation for this work (McLean and Andrew 2000).

Of note is that the reforms have tended to increase the numbers of children and families coming to the attention of child protection authorities, often due to risk-aversive approaches by governments and a belief that with further refinements and resources to the system, public confidence would be restored (CMC 2004; Lonne and Thomson 2005; Ainsworth and Hansen 2006; Mansell 2006b). These changes inevitably required more staff to meet the increased expectations of surveillance and investigation (Mansell 2006a), as well as the system requirements of greater data collection and input, and training in policies and procedures. At the same time, there has been a danger that many who might require help and intervention are never referred into the system or are quickly filtered out (Melton and Thompson 2002; Shireman 2003; Cooper *et al.* 2003; Pelton 2008)

More particularly, many governments have invested in children and there have been steady and sizeable increases in the budgetary allocations expended to herald these changes (Ainsworth and Hansen 2006; Parton 2006b), which have generally enjoyed widespread community and professional support (Mansell 2006b; E. Scott 2006). For example, the changes in Queensland, Australia following the Crime and Misconduct Commission's inquiry into foster care (CMC 2004) led to a tripling of the annual child protection budget to $531m within 4 years (Minister D. Boyle press release July 24, 2007). By anyone's terms these are sizeable fiscal commitments and belie the oft stated claim that governments are not prepared to invest in children and families. In fact, the size of budgetary increases to fund the escalating reports is arguably unsustainable (Ainsworth and Hansen 2006). Given that child protection systems experience chronic failure in the achievement of their missions (which are admittedly too broad), there is understandable annoyance on the part of political and bureaucratic figures that despite significant increases in scarce resources, the situation does not seem to improve, with ongoing system and practice failures evident. Rather, these fiscal escalations result in increased reports that only result in evermore strident calls for more money to relieve the stretched systems and overburdened staff. It is little wonder that such demand-driven systems are geared toward ongoing expansion and, further, are unable to be curtailed without fundamental reforms (Mansell 2006a,b). In short, they are unsustainable because they must eventually outstrip the capacity of governments to fund them, notwithstanding some evidence in the USA of recent plateauing in maltreatment and victimization levels (Finkelhor and Jones 2006). There have been other change management issues besides fiscal ones.

Taken overall, change management processes have often compounded the problems being experienced within these unsustainable systems and it is important to understand these in order to learn from them and minimize the likelihood of further complicating an ambitious reform agenda (Wells 2006). Melton and Thompson (2002) have argued that there is significant resistance to reforms within contemporary child protection systems, and that this is for reasons other than historical and administrative inertia. Change fatigue for staff who have experienced almost continual alterations to systems, policies and procedures compounds this resistance and needs to be taken into account when determining the pace of reform. It is essential to get staff on board with the need for, direction of, and steps required in, the reform agenda. The problems often experienced in change management of child protection have occurred at many levels and an examination of these can assist in developing appropriate strategies.

We have already established the extent to which child protection has become politicized (Cooper *et al.* 2003; Merrick 2006), often as a result of the desire by aspiring politicians to use the strident rhetoric of neoconservative and neoliberal ideologies in an effort to portray themselves as being pro-family and child-friendly. Unfortunately, the resultant political debate and hype around complex policy dilemmas and decisions has meant that reform processes have sometimes been at the mercy of changing political winds and clever but simplistic political catch cries that engender broad public and community support. Because reforms of the child protection system can be contentious among professional and community stakeholders, we argue that it is critical to have solid political support, and ideally for this to be across the political divides that exist. Our earlier point about the consensus that exists about improving protective systems is important, because this provides the mandate and platform for an effective change process. Reconfiguring the relationship between the state, families, parents, and children to become better aligned with enhancing well-being rather than just overt social surveillance requires broad political support to be successful.

A key failing of contemporary change management processes has resulted from attempts to assuage a multitude of claims makers and community stakeholders through making the organizational mission too broad and thereby unachievable. Because of the dominance of the child protection discourse and risk-aversive policy settings and organizational requirements, the result in many locations has been the continued ramping up of a forensic approach rather than a helping one, while in other locations, such as the UK, the discourse has been about prevention that also entails increased state intrusion into family life. These changes have been accompanied by two other powerful trends: a strengthening of managerialist power over professional knowledge-based power and an over-reliance on the development of ICT to provide up-to-date information on performance criteria and to solve communication problems both within and between agencies. These overall trends have often been associated with change leaders emphasizing a curbing of professional discretion and autonomy as well as compliance with policy and procedure rather than imprecise notions of sound social work practice (Froggett 2002; Wells 2006). The ICT explosion has also profoundly altered the professional role (Parton 2007) by elevating the tasks of data collection, in-putting and retrieval to key ones that significantly intrude on the time available to develop relationships with clients and assist them to change, a primary motivation for most helping professionals.

Compounding this has been a tendency for the imposition of top-down change management processes, and leadership approaches that have sometimes relied on coercive directives to staff to change or face the consequences—an uncanny parallel process with the ways in which parents and carers have sometimes felt they were treated by front-line staff (Smith and Donovan 2003; Dumbrill 2006). All too often this has been accompanied by a focus upon "accountability" which has been tantamount to blaming practitioners for system failures. This has often occurred with language that has portrayed political leaders and senior executives as valiant change agents trying to overcome social work incompetence on a grand scale—locating the problem squarely with professional social work rather than with identifying management or political leadership as part of the issue. The importance of the significant distinctions between the managerialist and professional discourses is noted here, with the former focusing on structural rearrangements and performance criteria that all too often are ideologically based within neoliberal ideologies, which run counter to the collective ideology implicit in social work (Froggett 2002). These NPM performance indicators are frequently narrowly defined and aligned to political imperatives rather than to real outcomes for children and families (Tilbury 2004, 2006). In short, management and staff have been speaking different languages (Lonne and Thomson 2005). Taken together, these broad trends have significantly contributed to a clear distancing and distrust in the relationships between management and front-line staff, and a tendency to undermine consensus about needed reform agendas, thereby thwarting well-intentioned and genuine efforts at change management.

The other notable failure of change management processes in many jurisdictions has been the general tendency to locate change management centrally within the child protection agency, sometimes to the exclusion of community-based issues and stakeholders. While the NPM and child protection discourses have embraced the importance of the language of "partnership," "collaboration," "consultation," and "community," there is scant evidence of this being translated into observable changes in the level of real participation of community within child protection systems. Melton and Thompson (2002) have identified that in the USA the major issue is neglect, mostly found in impoverished neighborhoods that have major social problems and little social capital, with there being a dire need to develop localized networks of informal assistance as well as formal helpers to create caring communities to promote economic and social development (Jack 2004; Hornberger and Briar-Lawson 2005).

Sadly, despite the rhetoric, child protection change management processes have generally given these goals a very low priority and have often been preoccupied with the internal machinations of developing sophisticated investigation systems that allow little meaningful ongoing participation and sharing of power by professional and community stakeholders (Melton and Thompson 2002). Consultations that do occur are often tokenistic and tend to be more about the agency telling others what it is intending to do, with power and control retained and even bolstered by a reluctance to fully inform external bodies about their intentions. Political and bureaucratic leaders have sometimes only reluctantly released their tight control of reform agendas, and there has been little opportunity for professional and community stakeholders to actively participate in the decision making about shaping system change. For example, linkages with educators and trainers of staff have been tenuous despite the clear need for newly trained professionals to have up-to-date knowledge of child protection policy and practices, as well as the requisite skills to enable them to form productive relationships with children and parents, and to deal with the stresses and strains of this work (Healy and Meagher 2007). Without community participating in, and being on side with, reform implementation processes the results are likely to be limited and may even be counterproductive to community capacity building (Froggett 2002; Melton and Thompson 2002; Jack 2004; Hornberger and Briar-Lawson 2005). We believe that the meaningful partnerships with professional and community stakeholders in the implementation of the reform agenda and the ongoing management of child protection, and child and family well-being programs, is critical to its success and ownership by the broad community.

Principles and themes for change management processes

Just as it is critically important not to adopt a "one size fits all" approach to reforming child protection and to understand the need to fit the reforms within the local context, so it is also necessary to match the general principles and themes of change management processes to the unique circumstances that one confronts. To successfully introduce and implement reform requires change leaders to have a very clear vision of the new system and how its values, structures, processes, policies, practices, and outcomes are interconnected. We also recognize that reform on the scale proposed will take time, and that development will be an iterative process, with time and space needed for reflexive analysis of the strategic directions and issues, the approaches being used, and the real outcomes that are eventuating. The embracing of reflective and reflexive practice by management and practice systems is an essential requirement if child protection and well-being systems are to make full use of their experiences, both positive and negative, to aid and guide their growth and development (Froggett 2002; Fook 2004). Effective professional (rather than administrative) supervision remains a central mechanism for promoting reflection and development. Effective change and reform require robust processes for systemic learning, and reflective practice is particularly useful in this regard.

We do not advocate introducing reforms with a "bang" as we believe that these sorts of approaches are often counterproductive in the longer term and can do great damage to individuals, groups and communities along the way, especially those who have legitimate viewpoints which are at variance to the "vision." Effective and beneficial change is built around convincing and inspiring people to embrace the vision, and to work hard on achieving regular progressive increments toward the desired goals. It is impossible to control all the processes and outcomes but, perhaps more importantly, it is ethically unsustainable to implement reform through employing power to overrule all opposition.

We hold to the notion of parallel processes in child protection systems: How management relates with and responds to staff can be replicated in psychodynamic ways with the ways in which practitioners then interact with service users. So adopting approaches that are power-laden, directive, and dismissive of others will be likely to result in poor processes and outcomes for children, parents and carers. Therefore, values-based leadership and management of personnel are critical. Leaders must "practice what they preach," as incongruence is apt to further attenuate management–staff relationships and hinder reform. Moreover, leaders who demonstrate behaviors and attitudes that are respectful and relationship-based are powerful role models for staff.

The themes and principles we believe are critical for successful reform processes include:

• embracing an ethical and positive value framework for management and practice (e.g. respect, care, virtuous);
• modeling leadership that is practice-informed, engaged, listening, and dialogue-oriented, open to alternative perspectives, and able to articulate and inspire people with the vision for reform;
• holding to a clear vision of the required outcomes of change while being flexible in exactly how and when structural alterations and other strategies are implemented to achieve the reforms;
• utilizing a range of communication processes and forums to ensure that diverse professional and community stakeholders are kept informed of developments, and engaged in debates about the issues and options;
• proactively promoting the active participation of community stakeholders in the management of implementing the reform agenda at all levels;
• managing the change processes in transparent and truly accountable ways;
• employing contemporary management tools and processes to plan, implement, monitor, and review progress without letting these and the associated discourse dominate over the practice discourse; and
• embracing reflective practice as a cornerstone of management and professional practice in order to learn effectively from review, monitoring, and modification processes.

We emphasize the critical role of proactive leadership at the political, organizational, professional, practice, neighborhood, and community levels. Without courageous, inspiring and committed leadership it will be difficult, if not impossible, to overcome the systemic inertia that can thwart reform. Great leaders take people with them: sometimes taking charge and leading from the front, and sometimes following the collective view of others. We have used the term "practice-informed" in a broad sense and see it as utilizing knowledge of professional practice and child protection (see Turnell and Edwards 1999), as well as skills such as understanding group and organizational dynamics, using power and authority appropriately, sensitively managing the politics, and being able to balance appropriately the need to direct, guide and coordinate people in change processes. This involves respecting others, communicating clearly, dialoguing effectively, influencing and inspiring others, delegating appropriately, and making tough decisions when needed.

Management of reform also requires knowledge or organizational, program and community development principles and processes. Change is rarely straightforward and does not always go according to plan. It is fluid, messy and uncertain with progress being variable and the steps being non-linear and sometimes unexpected, even sideways or backwards. Good managers know this and have the skills to be able to respond flexibly in principled and planned ways that progresses the change agenda, while continuing to stay well connected with stakeholders. Virtue ethics entails demonstrating personal qualities such as treating others fairly and justly, displaying loyalty and trust in the roles of others, and acting reflectively, prudently, and with integrity (Froggett 2002; McBeath and Webb 2002). These approaches are necessary if people are to develop confidence in the change management directions and processes.

Good stewardship of resources is also critical, but can be difficult because of the demand issues that we highlighted earlier and the resultant effects on reports and service delivery (Shireman 2003; Mansell 2006a,b). We posit that a system as we have suggested will attend to this critical issue through specific measures that ensure decision making about reports is in keeping with restricted legislative definitions and heightened emphasis on the rights of families to privacy considerations. From our viewpoint, there is a rapidly growing groundswell of stakeholders across Anglophone countries who are deeply troubled by the poor outcomes being achieved for a range of people with current approaches to the protection of children, and wish dearly for profound system change. We will now touch upon how their common interest in seeing how a better system can be harnessed to achieve this.

Systemic change processes

There are many stakeholders with sometimes diverse interests and viewpoints who must contribute to bring to fruition the reform of child protection. Differences in views reflect moral, political (sexuality, family, roles, status, gender) and scientific issues and can go across usual political leanings (Mildred 2003). Bringing these stakeholders together to support reform is challenging and requires considerable commitment but, in our view, is achievable because all share in a desire to have a system that is fair and just, and which protects the vulnerable and addresses the social care needs of individuals and the broad community. The vision for reform must be communicated unambiguously and in a straightforward fashion so that everyone is clear about the direction being taken and the changes necessary to achieve it.

Our vision is for a comprehensive system of integrated agencies and processes that build child and family well-being, foster helping and caring connections between people, and thereby develop safer, healthier, and more sustaining neighborhoods and communities. Service delivery is accessible, needs-focused, relationship-based, and ethical (Turnell and Edwards 1999; Froggett 2002), with an emphasis on addressing the individual, family, neighborhood, community, and societal factors that contribute to abuse and neglect of children (Melton and Thompson 2002; Freymond and Cameron 2006). Agencies need to be embedded within communities and neighborhoods, and values should drive practice that is built on collaborative helping relation-ships. Moreover, practice and policy must not resile from affording vulnerable children and families the protection and opportunities they need, while also articulating clear expectations of safety and care (Turnell and Edwards 1999).

There are many processes involved in bringing about policy change and systemic reform. First, it is necessary to problematize the current situation and arrangements by identifying issues that are perceived by government and/or community stakeholders as "problems" and requiring a policy response. This is a process of social construction that involves taking ideological positions, making decisions based on social beliefs and values, and prioritizing goals and objectives (Cheers *et al.* 2007). While there are many critics of current approaches to protecting children, a key aspect of the change process is prioritizing these different goals and objectives.

According to Bridgman and Davis (2004), in the second phase of the policy process, the bureaucracy analyzes the presenting issues and factors influencing them, and develops rationales for action, including selecting policy instruments (e.g., legislation and service programs). This is followed by consultation with selected stakeholders, inside and external to government, with clear social policy options generated. Government then makes decisions and resources programs to address the issues at hand, these being implemented with outcomes being evaluated, leading to a re-examination of the issues. Policy production is instrumental and authoritative in this framework, politicians making the final determinations, while the public sector tends to the administrative func-tions. Brodkin (2000) calls this approach "command-and-control" because political and administrative authorities use their power to include or exclude input from specific stakeholders. Sadly, contemporary child protection policy making typically adopts these sorts of orthodox approaches, thereby excluding many stakeholders, particularly children and parents, from finding voice and influence.

Moreover, in our view, while this circular process is a useful conceptual framework, it belies the inherent uncertainty, unpredictability, ambiguity, complexity, and disorder in policy processes. There are numerous decision makers involved in child and family policy, and among the different stake-holders competition and contestability of advice abound. No single authorita-tive voice on any particular child welfare issue is found. "Rather, there are a multitude of voices that compete or collaborate with each other, some of which are powerful and influential while others are not" (Cheers *et al.* 2007: 34). However, this complex and fluid process, influenced by the erratic nature of politics, nevertheless provides many opportunities for the community, other stakeholders, managers, and practitioners to influence policy making, some-times despite the endeavors of political and bureaucratic authorities. An example of this policy-making dynamism is the sometimes large-scale change that occurs as a result of catastrophic events such as child deaths, although it must be noted that the risk-averse political and organizational cultures often result in counterproductive reforms occurring (Munro 2004b; Lonne and Thomson 2005; Connolly and Doolan 2006, 2007). When there is a chorus of clamoring calls for practitioner "culprits" to be named and shamed and demands for no child to ever be harmed, it can be very difficult for the voice of reason to be heard (Connolly and Doolan 2006, 2007; D. Scott 2006a), particularly when reports rise dramatically (Mansell 2006a,b). At times like these, strong and effective leadership holds firm and re-articulates the vision as well as responding in calm and measured ways to accountability needs. Good policy rarely comes from panic-driven responses to incidents of bad practice.

Nevertheless, these tragic events do provide an opening for debate and dialogue about the systemic issues plaguing child protection, and help to build a groundswell for the need for change. We believe that there is a critical need for influential stakeholders, including the media, to build the pressure for change until it is irresistible. Groups such as those representing children and families who come into contact with the child protection system, professional associations and practitioner unions, academics and researchers, need to mobilize into coalitions to both inform the debates and present different approaches and options. This book provides clear policy and structural options to provide a pathway for reform. In doing this, it offers positive alternatives to those typically put forward in the sometimes ill-informed and knee-jerk reactions that seek to blame and punish, and to make the system even more proceduralized, managerialized, and regulated (Froggett 2002; Connolly and Doolan 2006, 2007).

We assert that the broad public wants a system that is fair and just, and which will provide a web of assistance and protection to vulnerable children and families. Politicians are critical allies in the pursuit of systemic and policy change, not least because of their public leadership roles and their ability to harness the attention of the media and other communication forums that tap into, as well as reflect, the community concerns and aspirations. While we acknowledge that politicians have sometimes spearheaded the race to have audit, accountability, proceduralism, and blaming as characteristics of contemporary systems, we also recognize that many politicians have also been the voice of reason when some others have called for "heads to roll." In either event, large-scale systemic and policy change does not usually occur unless there are influential political figures championing the need for change and the vision of a better alternative. Hence, alliances and coalitions between stakeholder groups and politicians is a necessary step in reforming child protection. Politicians can help overcome the inertia that hinders systemic change.

People who are not used to playing community leadership and political roles are sometimes reluctant to become involved, being unsure of the processes and requirements, and possibly fearing the implications of failure. However, systems theory alerts us that small change can potentially have profound effects on a bigger system and lead to seismic shifts in policy and structures—"out of little things big things grow." We outlined earlier how carer and workforce issues abound within these systems. Significant dissatisfaction is felt by these key stakeholders and they can be major players in leading system reform. Staff and carers know the shortcomings in resources and service delivery standards because they experience them daily. They appreciate the inherent complexities but also the degree of personal pain felt by children and families who seek an end to the abuse and neglect, and help to change their circumstances for the better.

Children and families who come into contact with child protection systems themselves are critically important to the sort of change required. We acknowledge their relative powerlessness within these systems and, particularly for parents, the public labelling and condemnation they frequently receive. Nevertheless, they remain central figures in the change process because their experiences provide compelling examples of both what can happen to assist people to change their lives as well as what should not happen. For example, an Australian mother whose toddler recently died from injuries allegedly received from his father, expressed her grief and concern about the child protection intervention that was provided—"The person who is working with you doesn't know the situation. The Department . . . change their case workers like they change their frigging underpants" (*Sunday Mail* 2007). The mother claimed that despite her son being under a statutory protection order, departmental officers had not responded to her calls for help a month earlier. These sorts of stories are heard all too often. They depict contemporary systems as being largely unable to provide the sort of help required to address the safety and other issues, sometimes with tragic consequences.

We have argued for a broad range of community stakeholders and, in particular, children, parents and caregivers to have far greater input into policy processes and organizations so that community needs, aspirations and contexts are incorporated into service delivery structures and processes, and that social capital is built (Froggett 2002). For too long child protection systems have been detached and remote from local neighborhoods and communities, practicing on them rather than within them (Melton and Thompson 2002; Cooper *et al.* 2003; Jack 2004; Hornberger and Briar-Lawson 2005; Freymond and Cameron 2006). We believe that the power imbalances between these stakeholders and child welfare authorities need to be addressed in a number of ways, including structurally through the creation of local Community Child and Family Well-being Boards. These can play a critical role in over-seeing the implementation of reforms, and system processes and outcomes. They can provide invaluable feedback and guidance about how best to implement programs and deliver services because they involve broad-based linkages with community. Hence, they offer an important feedback loop which can inform change management along the way and monitor the real impacts of change. Moreover, they will help build trust and cooperation in broader system relations.

Collectively, all these stakeholder groups have contact with the managers and executives who hold organizational responsibility and authority for policy and operations, and who have the ability to change the system. Indeed, the numerous reforms that have already occurred (albeit unsuccessfully) have largely been driven by senior staff. We therefore reject the sometimes simplistic media analyses that blame management and depict them as the root causes for all the problems we have outlined. Many factors have been at play and to single out one group for responsibility is unfair and unhelpful. We see managers and executives as important people to have on side because they will implement and steer the reform process.

Organizational change management processes

Management plays a key leadership role necessary to bring about effective change processes that result in agency and systemic reform. While leadership is demonstrated by staff at all levels, dynamic senior executives and politicians are critical if a broad consensus about the reform vision and agenda is to emerge. The complex and fluid social policy-making processes in Anglophone countries involve important parts being played by a large range of government and community stakeholders, in particular executive management of central government departments. Legislative, policy, and systemic change entails a substantial redirection of government priorities and approaches and has to be cast in the language of "reform" so that key organizational decision makers will embrace and champion it (Diefenbach 2007).

But politicians, executives and managers can also be resistant to change and sometimes play significant parts in maintaining administrative inertia (Melton and Thompson 2002). This may stem from inadequate resourcing and not having the organizational wherewithal to embark upon substantive reform (Shireman 2003), preferring resistance or incremental change. Sometimes, in an effort to deal with community complaints and media criticisms (which can be unfair and unbalanced), some child protection agencies develop an organizational culture and climate that is defensive, closed, and tantamount to "bunkering down" under sustained attack. This sensitivity to criticism and defensiveness can prevent organizations from self-reflection and development processes that are needed to effect change. Those agitating for change can sometimes become despondent and disillusioned when their energetic efforts and representations "fall on deaf ears." Further blaming is frequently counterproductive and just increases the level of resistance.

Instead, our suggestion is to work with people in an effort to build the coalitions and trust that are necessary to establish a shared understanding of the impetus and urgency for change. This entails recognizing and giving support to the many genuine efforts to change and reform. Without political and bureaucratic support, change of the current system is very difficult indeed. Conversely, once there is substantial organizational support for system change, there is a powerful flow-on effect across government and community organizations that is impossible to ignore and difficult to resist (Cheers *et al.* 2007). Community stakeholders therefore play an important role in building and sustaining the change management processes, particularly in their ability to support those in leadership roles with guidance rather than criticisms that offer no helpful and do-able alternatives. Further, it is important for community stakeholders to understand the complex processes that change management involves and have realistic expectations of what can be achieved in the short and medium terms (Nunno 2006).

A useful framework for government and external stakeholders to understand organizational reform processes such as those we advocate is provided by Kotter (2007). Center stage in this framework is the vision, which we have detailed in the preceding chapters, but also important are creating alliances within and external to the organization, empowering people to implement the vision, and using planning and review mechanisms to embed the changes. We note the criticality of reflective practice in assisting professional social care practitioners to develop their knowledge, skills and wisdom (Froggett 2002). Kotter's (2007) eight aspects of successful change processes include:

1   Establishing a great enough sense of urgency
2   Creating a powerful guiding coalition
3   Creating a vision
4   Communicating the vision
5   Empowering others to act on the vision and removing obstacles
6   Planning for and creating short term wins
7   Consolidating improvements and producing more change, and
8   Institutionalizing new approaches.

Kotter highlights the importance of having a central champion of change who can not only clearly articulate the vision and the desired goals and objectives, but also the need to assemble allies who share the vision into a powerful force for change at multiple levels of the organization and externally. Importantly, change management should be grounded and attend to obstacles that arise as well as ensuring that milestones are achieved regularly, thereby demonstrating success. We emphasize the criticality of having dynamic change management leadership at the executive level.

However, middle managers and front-line staff also have critical roles because they manage the interfaces between the macro policy settings and resources, neighborhood and community contexts, organizational cultures and climates, and service delivery and workgroup issues (Brodkin 2000). We firmly believe that addressing the human resource issues that abound in contemporary child protection systems is an important starting point in change management, because without capable, committed and intuitive professional staff who demonstrate wisdom, changing the nature of worker–client relationships will be difficult if not impossible (Turnell and Edwards 1999; Froggett 2002). Professional supervision must be a primary mechanism for achieving these sorts of practice transformations. Bednar (2003) notes that: "ideally, the role of the supervisor in such a system would be supportive and consultative, and would enable direct-service staff to engage in self-actualizing work with clients" (p. 11). Trust in staff is essential to enlist them into the vision and the reform process and thereby reshape their relationships with service users, other stakeholders, and the community (Froggett 2002; Cooper *et al.* 2003; Smith and Donovan 2003). Rebuilding the child and family well-being workforce necessitates addressing the chronic recruitment problems, reducing staff turnover to acceptable levels, providing a satisfying work environment where staff are respected, supportively supervised, well trained, and able to respond effectively to diverse client needs, and establishing policy and practice frameworks where effective staff–client relationships can be developed (Savicki 2002; Shireman 2003).

Great strides have been made in some locations demonstrating that these issues can be remedied. For example, by using the ARC interventions to address organizational climate and related issues in a Tennessee USA child welfare agency, staff turnover was reduced by two-thirds, and staff reported reduced role conflict, role overload, emotional exhaustion and depersonal- ization (Glisson *et al.* 2006). The flow-on effects to service delivery outcomes and inter-agency coordination were significant, with effective casework relationships being "more likely to occur where caseworkers agree on their roles, are satisfied with their jobs, cooperate with each other, and personalize their work" (Glisson and Hemmelgarn 1998: 404–5). Many child protection agencies are developing innovative staff support capabilities, such as the Department of Child Safety in Queensland Australia (2006), which has created a range of programs to address factors affecting stress and staff turnover. Being responsive to the needs of staff is a critical step in improving service delivery, because of the parallel processes we described earlier. When staff are respected and valued by management they are well placed to treat children, parents, and carers in a similar fashion. Robust professional supervision is the key. Therefore, values-based HRM and leadership are required.

Changing organizational climate and cultures is difficult in contemporary managerialized and proceduralized child protection systems where "pressures from an institutionalized environment hinder the use of client-centered, strength-based practices" (Smith and Donovan 2003: 561–2). However, where there are clear visions for a better future, sufficient resources, and the drive and commitment from management and staff, great things can happen. Enlisting staff who may be "change fatigued" into reform processes is not necessarily easy, and requires management to use a practice-oriented discourse, rather than one that is located solely within contemporary NPM. We do not suggest that business practices such as strategic planning and review, mission statements, business plans, and performance/outcome indicators are, in them- selves, problematic. Indeed, the sort of structural and policy reforms that we have outlined in this book require robust planning and change manage- ment approaches to assist in coordinating an ambitious series of changes.

Rather, we suggest that there are major problems when NPM is used to devalue the professional discourse, disempower staff and reorient the focus of social welfare policy away from helping to address social care needs into purely punitive systems of surveillance and social control. Unfortunately, this is the situation in many child protection systems.

Managers need to be practice-informed leaders of people who can coordinate planning and operations and, importantly, embrace openness and accountability, for this is what they expect of front-line staff. In contemporary vernacular they must "talk the talk and walk the walk." Highly developed communication skills are essential, including the ability to relate to and communicate with a diverse range of people with respect, sincerity and appropriate use of authority. Because there is always an element of conflict in child welfare work, all staff must be able to effectively manage and, where possible, resolve this (Turnell and Edwards 1999). Leadership qualities necessary for people at all levels include being able to dialogue with and listen to others, treating them fairly and justly, using power and authority appropriately, and displaying loyalty, trust, and confidence. When managers treat staff in these ways they are able to influence and inspire them to achieve collective goals. This places them in a good position to effectively communicate the vision, facilitate goal achievement, manage resources and improve performance.

To transition practice a heavy emphasis is needed upon retraining staff to ensure that the values and approaches we describe are embraced at all levels, so that they can work effectively with children, families, carers, and other stakeholders. The training should focus on relationship-based practice and how this is used as the vehicle to assist children and families to make the changes necessary to prevent abuse and neglect. Professional supervision and reflective practice also need to be actively promoted to develop practitioners' skills and knowledge. As practitioners, researchers, and educators, we believe that there is a critical need to develop closer working relationships and linkages with universities, other educators, and professional associations to ensure that the right knowledge and skill set is emphasized and developed. Unfortunately, too often there has been a separation between what students are taught and the knowledge and skills requirements of what is exceptionally complex work (Healy and Meagher 2007). Professional associations can be valuable allies for reform, by highlighting and articulating the need for change, and emphasizing ethical and professional practice standards, and social policy viewpoints.

We emphasize that planning and preparation are the keys to successful implementation. Too often, change in child protection and child welfare agencies occurs as a reactive consequence of tragedies or scandals, and the political imperative to change quickly leaves managers with an impossible task that has adverse consequences for staff and service users. Successful change management and program implementation are also fundamentally reliant upon structured review and evaluation processes, where information is collated, analyzed and used to inform and guide ongoing development. Mindful of the shortcomings in child protection system performance indicators that Tilbury (2004, 2005, 2006) identified, we advocate for holistic qualitative and quantitative performance and change indicators to be used so that the real outcomes for children, families and the broad community are identified. Client-focused evaluations are necessary for they can provide greater awareness and understanding of the lived experiences of those who require assistance. Detailed information on how people's lives are affected must drive policy and service delivery approaches. Client-focused evaluation and research is essential to gauge the extent of cultural and practice change, and to measure and analyze the effects of the shifts in policy and the processes used to change organizational cultures and practices.

Given the chequered career of previous policy and structural changes in child protection and child welfare systems, the pervasive influence of NPM, and the adverse impacts of risk-averse and audit-driven practice, we have advocated for significant structural, policy, and practice reforms. The implementation of large-scale systemic reforms is rarely, if ever, straightforward and we do not suggest it will be problem-free. There is a need to wisely use robust strategic and business planning and review processes in order to minimize the likelihood of experiencing major implementation issues, and to incorporate evaluative and reflective practice mechanisms to ensure that valuable learnings are not passed by. The collaborative involvement of children, parents, caregivers, staff, and other stakeholders from the community within the management and implementation processes is integral to a well functioning child and family well-being system that is accessible and beneficial to those in need. An ethical, values- and relationship-based system is more likely than current approaches to provide safety, security, help, and guidance to those in need, and thereby promote child and family, and community well-being.

Part 4

Crisis? What crisis?

The past and the future:
choice and chance

10 Change and the future of child and family well-being practice

In this book we have undertaken three tasks essential for systemic change. First, we have provided an evidence-based critique of contemporary Anglophone child protection systems and their outcomes in relation to service users and stakeholders. We then outlined a vision for a better approach to responding to the complex problems of child abuse and neglect, including practice principles, an ethical and values-based framework, along with altered structural and practice arrangements. In doing this we have used the concept of child and family well-being to describe a reformed system that rebalances the social care and social control functions, and is reoriented toward ethical relationships as a key mechanism for influencing families to change and develop. Finally, we described how to manage and undertake these changes, mindful of the enormity of the change management processes required and the potential effects on child protection systems that have, in most cases, been subject to rapid and ongoing modifications to their functions and operations for many years.

Our intention has been to establish a compelling case for change by highlighting the limitations and failures of the current constructions of, and approaches to, child protection in Anglophone countries, and to suggest that, taken overall, these systems hurt more people than they help. Fundamental change is therefore required. Our analysis goes beyond narrow audits that focus on individual actions to instead examine how these systems work as a whole and the outcomes they achieve overall. We do not wish to continue the counterproductive "blame game" of seeking out those who are deemed accountable, according to them responsibility for the failures that are largely structurally and systemically based. Conversely, we believe that these systems rely upon the commitment, skills, courage and strength of character of a myriad of dedicated staff at all levels in order to make them work, and that they undertake this work in child protection systems which are underpinned by punitive ideologies and technologies. Without the steadfast and difficult work undertaken by such staff the situation would be far worse. Moreover, we argue that these good staff are the cornerstone of the efforts required to address the problems and effect systemic change.

We acknowledge the limitations of language in our endeavors to critique contemporary practices and reform child protection. Similar terms can mean very different things to different people, the term "child abuse" being a clear example. There are diverse social constructions of the terms used to describe the phenomenon of child abuse and neglect, dependent upon factors such as culture, gender, and community location, and the historical and organizational cultural contexts within different agencies. In writing about child protection systems across different countries, locations, and cultural groupings there will inevitably be potential for misunderstandings as to exact meanings, particularly when system and research data and findings are examined. Definitional imprecision is typical, with a variety of approaches taken, and meanings adopted, in determining system and outcome indicators. Hence, when we compare child protection data including reports, investigation outcomes, and intervention responses we find that substantial differences in terminology make it problematic to compare systems. Despite these inherent limitations, comparisons across jurisdictions are vitally important as they allow us to examine and evaluate different approaches and interventions, and thereby understand how people across jurisdictions are grappling with the complexity found in preventing, and intervening in, situations that harm children.

We also acknowledge the limitations in our attempts to find a common language in this book that accurately captures the key points as well as the similarities and differences apparent across Anglophone countries, communities, cultures, and child protection jurisdictions. For example, while we know that there is considerable difference in the legislation and operational practices within Australian state government jurisdictions, there is also significant similarity of the models of intervention (Bromfield and Higgins 2005). Similarly, there is much diversity in child protection practice in the USA, but taken overall, there are many similarities as well. While we have sought, where appropriate, to draw generalized conclusions in order to highlight macro contexts and dynamics, we have also used specific examples to highlight particular situations and points, and thereby illustrate the diversity that exists.

Recognizing the diversity is important because it allows consideration of the more generalized as well as the specific contexts in which reform and change agendas are played out and operationalized. While we have offered a range of reform proposals, we understand that analysis of the specific local community and organizational contexts is required along with modifications of our suggestions in order for them to be congruent with the unique situations that present within individual jurisdictions. Hence, we are not suggesting that our proposals should be slavishly adhered to or that they will suit every community context. Rather, we recommend that the relevance and merit of our critiques of contemporary approaches and the principles, values, and structural alterations that we suggest should be critically examined so that culturally appropriate applications of the reform agenda can be undertaken.

In this sense we are not suggesting our proposals should be prescriptive and universally applied. Rather, we suggest that they provide options for responses that will address the major issues that confront us regarding the processes and outcomes of child protection as it is practiced in many, but not all, communities in Anglophone countries. Our suggested reforms can be seen as important contributions to the debates which are currently occurring in academic, organizational, community, and governmental forums about the efficacy of current systems. Through dialogue and open discussion, and a preparedness to critically examine the current situation and identify its strengths, successes and failings, we will be able to explore conceptual and practical solutions to the problems that confront us.

As longstanding committed advocates for children, we have embarked on the journey of reform knowing that it is a long and arduous task that may involve many unforeseen pitfalls and hurdles. Nevertheless, we are resolute in our conviction that current approaches are failing and by any reasonable measure do not meet the needs, hopes, and aspirations of any of the stakeholders who are involved. For example:

- Children remain largely unheard and excluded from playing a robust part in systems that are established to further their interests and enhance their well-being.
- Children in care generally experience deplorable life outcomes.
- Many parents feel judged, punished and excluded by child protection processes and interventions, and are therefore less inclined to be positively motivated to make changes in their behavior and lives.
- Foster and alternative carers are often left to deal with very difficult and complex situations with little support and reward.
- Front-line staff typically endure organizational environments that are injurious to their long-term health and well-being.
- Managers, executives, and politicians are exasperated by the seemingly intractable difficulties in trying to rectify the shortcomings found in their organizations and service delivery outcomes.
- Communities are left feeling bewildered and outraged at the apparent inability of the organizations they entrust to protect children from abuse and neglect or assist struggling families who need help.

Before we re-examine the types of reforms that we have suggested, it is timely to revisit the evidence-based arguments outlined in the first half of this book in order to reacquaint ourselves with the complexities of current approaches, and to examine why they are not proving to be efficacious in addressing and preventing abuse and neglect that is occurring in our neighborhoods and communities.

The successes and failures of child protection

The history of child protection is a chequered one, with great successes achieved such as bringing the issues of abuse and neglect of children into the mainstream of community responses and governmental social policy initiatives, initially as part of a "child saving" approach but, increasingly over time, as a much broader and more sophisticated range of preventative and tertiary interventions into the lives of vulnerable children and families. The development of an elaborate network of social agencies into whole-of-government and, arguably, whole-of-community responses has occurred due to the hard work of committed child advocates who have raised the consciousness of Anglophone and other societies in regard to the needs and rights of children, viewing these as both congruent with, and also separate to, the needs and rights of parents, carers, and adults. It is now an exception rather than a rule to have adults who do not recognize the significance and scope of child abuse and neglect, and who support the obligation of the broad community to intervene to protect vulnerable children. It is self-evident that direct intervention by child protection authorities has meant that a large number of children and families have been protected, helped, and rescued from intolerable and unacceptable situations where abuse and neglect have hurt, humiliated, and damaged them and their relations with each other. However, these systems have also had a history of struggling to meet societal expectations and to provide the necessary help and guidance to vulnerable children and families that their mandate requires. We have noted also the significance of the iatrogenesis in these interventions, that is, their negative consequences for a number of stakeholders, including children.

Numerous iterations over the past two decades or more have occurred in the development of child welfare organizations, which subsequently transformed into child protection systems as we see them today. These changes occurred as a result of increased understandings of the nature and causes of abuse and neglect, as well as altered social mandates heralded by new legislative and policy frameworks. And they reflected and embraced the increasing social conservatism that characterized the prevailing ideologies found in Anglophone countries in the latter part of the twentieth century. For example, social policy was increasingly fashioned around neoliberal orientations toward governance and social relations, with economic and fiscal policies being driven by market-based imperatives and a reduced role for the state in determining how economies would function.

While there were some significant exceptions, taken overall, these policy shifts witnessed increasingly punitive approaches with emphasis upon individual responsibility and a downplaying of the influence of structural causes of social problems such as poverty and crime. While these broad trends were characteristic, there were nevertheless important differences found among Anglophone and other countries (McDonald *et al.* 2003; Khoo *et al.* 2002). Social welfare in general was seen as counterproductive to both macroeconomic efforts as well as to individuals, who were seen to be better off relying on their own resources rather than becoming dependent upon the state (McDonald 2006). The state became harsher in its orientation toward groups that were seen as dangerous, troublesome, or lazy, with social programs increasingly utilizing restrictive and punitive measures to control behavior deemed antisocial.

Parallel with these broad changes was a gradual escalation in an emphasis on social control in child protection policy and legislation, along with a more prominent role for police in the investigation of offences against children. Politicians frequently reacted to widespread community concerns about protecting children and scandals such as high profile child deaths by widening the definitional criteria in legislative and policy frameworks, with the broader concept of "harm," for example, replacing definitions of abuse and neglect. Over time, the net was widened considerably. The overall effect of these alterations was increased community awareness and heightened anxiety about the effects of not protecting children from abuse and neglect, and thereby increased demand for resources to deal with the problem. In nearly all jurisdictions there were exponential increases in the numbers of child abuse reports and by the 1990s these were placing severe strain on the ability of child protection agencies to undertake the necessary investigations and assessments of children deemed at risk.

This situation became unsustainable and led to one of the most profound of many subsequent systemic changes in policy—the advent of differential response, a process for assessing the relative risk to children and culling out low risk allegations by either providing advice to those notifying authorities of their concerns or the referral of the matter to voluntary and community-based family support agencies. However, as systems became larger and more complex to manage, cases were still able to slip between the different organizational responses. For example, Victoria Climbié in England was killed despite the involvement of a number of statutory agencies. Most importantly, she had been defined as a child in need of support rather than a child in need of protection. These tragedies further escalated demands for even tighter systems of surveillance so that no child would suffer such a terrible fate. Subsequently, the child protection system has become a giant surveillance and screening system in which practitioners trawl through floods of calls and reports from concerned citizens in the belief that this will successfully prevent further tragedies. In most, but not all, jurisdictions the result is a system dominated by forensic investigation and yet unable to provide effective help to the vulnerable and those in need, particularly children in care.

Moreover, child protection systems became increasingly reliant upon sophisticated information technology systems for the collation and analysis of client-related records and data. Backed by legislative requirements such as mandatory reporting and inter-agency protocols for information sharing, child protection practice developed enhanced surveillance capabilities not just over individuals, but also over particular groups such as women, single parents, and Indigenous peoples who tended to come to their notice more than other groups. As the child protection discourse overtook the child welfare or well-being discourse, so too did a tendency toward media demonizing of parents who abused or neglected their children. There is evidence to indicate that, at least to some extent, child protection policies have had different impacts on different groups of people. In this sense, while child abuse and neglect can occur in every section of society, child protection systems tended to keep their gaze squarely on particular groups who were characterized by increased "risk factors"—the advent of the "risk society" was to have a significant influence upon shaping child protection policy, procedure, and practice.

Throughout these iterations in the development of child protection the voices of service users, as well as other community-based stakeholders, have been largely unheard. Political and organizational agendas have tended to marginalize and ignore children, and demonize or ostracize parents, while child protection practitioners have either been put on a pedestal or blamed for system failings and tragedies. We suggest that through listening to these people affected by current approaches, and hearing their experiences, we can be better informed as to the intended and unintended consequences of these interventions into family lives. Just as service user voices have shaped contemporary mental health and disability services and practices, so too should they influence child protection. The voices of staff must also be heard. Far too many agencies turn a deaf ear to the pleas of front-line practitioners about the harm from organizational cultures and climates on their well-being. If committed staff would rather leave their jobs than remain on the front-line helping and protecting children, the system becomes unsustainable, because it relies upon their skills, knowledge, and involvement to facilitate positive changes in the lives of children, parents, and families.

Unfortunately, in response to scandals and other tragic events, formal inquiries have too often handed down narrow prescriptions for increased procedures to minimize the risk of mistakes, and audit functions to examine events, identify those at fault, and increase accountability, if not in individuals, then in systems. But in a paradoxical fashion, these approaches to treating the inherently risky business of child abuse and neglect, and the complexities in its prevention and interventions into family life, mostly complicated further the practice of child protection practitioners, leading to increased wariness to take risks of any sort that could "come back at them." The end result has often been risk-averse organizational environments and professional practice that has seen the unnecessary removal of children without full and proper assessment in too many cases (false positives), or the inadequate intervention to protect children who have been seriously abused and who required significant state involvement to ensure their safety and well-being (false negatives).

It is little wonder that in such strained and complex environments the need for robust management became increasingly apparent. As the reformation of social welfare came to pass in the latter half of the twentieth century, so did NPM with the benefits of managerialism promoted widely as an effective way of dealing with the problems of administering social policy and also of implementing change management agendas. It was often sold on claims that its emphasis on strategic review and planning, clear lines of managerial control, efficiency, performance management, and accountability mechanisms would fundamentally reform out-dated and ineffective approaches to public administration. But NPM did far more than this. With its attendant discourse based solidly on traditional management approaches, there was a large-scale shift in power and authority away from professional staff toward management, who were portrayed as having the answers to complex problems of how to "manage with less" and to implement the necessary accountability and efficiency regimes that would enable governments to implement their priorities.

Along with a host of other social policy program areas, such as education and health, child protection systems undertook a welter of reforms and modifications to policy under the guidance and control of managers whose preoccupation was less that of client-focused outcomes than system-focused ones. The language of risk, audit, accountability, performance, and managerial oversight predominated, arguably at the expense of traditional professional discourses that emphasized client outcomes, albeit within approaches that mostly embraced professional authority, power, and control.

A key mechanism for this transition from traditional casework approaches to service delivery was case management, which sought to implement more regimented and accountable frameworks for the structuring and delivery of social programs and services that would ensure service eligibility assessments and rationing of services in line with policy and budgetary priorities. Professional assessments and the relationship-based practice of traditional social work and other occupational groups were largely displaced. Based around policy and procedural requirements and performance standards and indicators, case management re-fashioned the nature of relationships between human service workers and service users. In child protection systems, case management was integral to the increased utilization of information and communication technologies as tools for the tracking, surveillance, and management of individuals and groups within policy frameworks.

It is apparent from the literature and research that the general nature of social relations between child protection practitioners and service users altered to become more power-laden and controlling. In this sense there was a parallel process between the ways in which front-line staff often perceived they were treated by management systems, and the ways in which service users often felt they were dealt with by front-line staff. The shifts toward social control at the expense of social care, as well as the increased incidence of threats and violence toward staff, have probably contributed to the unsustainably high rates of work-related stress and staff turnover. Committed staff have been "voting with their feet" and, in some jurisdictions, resultant recruitment difficulties have meant that there has been immense pressures on organizations to lower professional educational requirements in order to recruit sufficient staff to address the workload. This de-professionalization places further pressure on already struggling systems and on the service delivery standards that are necessary to meet their societal mandates and organizational missions.

To our way of thinking, the history of child protection demonstrates significant successes on a number of fronts and there is no doubt that programs focusing on the needs and safety of children are essential in any civil society. However, despite these successes, the shortcomings and limitations of emergent Anglophone child protection systems remain clearly evident and indicate that current approaches are often counterproductive to the safety and well-being of too many children, parents and families. We believe that, over time, the almost constant legislative, organizational, and program changes that have occurred within child protection systems have rendered them less capable of meeting their central task of protecting vulnerable children and families, particularly children who are in care. Moreover, the system dynamics are such as to make many agencies unsustainable and in urgent need of fundamental reforms. In making this case, we acknowledge that the seriousness of the current situation means that change must occur at a number of levels and that further reforms will put these systems under increased pressure. Nevertheless, change they must, or risk ongoing failure to meet the needs of children and families for safety, security, and well-being.

The reform agenda

Practice principles

In formulating our ideas for this book calling for reform of child protection systems, we explored the history of almost continual systemic changes and why these had largely been unsuccessful, and sometimes counterproductive to their broad social mandate. As longstanding and committed child advocates, we reached a collective conclusion that further modification at the edges was not helpful and may make things worse. Rather, we determined that fundamental reforms of the ethics, practice, organizations, and other structures are urgently required. We are not alone in reaching this position (Cooper *et al.* 2003; Melton 2005; D. Scott 2006a; Pelton 2008). Many practitioners, researchers and academics across Anglophone countries have also expressed deep reservations about the current state of affairs. Collectively, child advocates need to have the courage of their convictions when identifying the sorts of systemic failings we have outlined. Highlighting that our systems are not working is a critical first step in the change process that leads to broader reform. However, we wanted this book to offer more than just a critique of the current system, and opted for a clear proposal of how a new approach to child and family well-being might look. Our alternative system includes guiding principles, ethical and practice frameworks, and altered structural arrangements for service delivery and community participation.

Recent events at the US Transportation Security Administration (TSA) provide a powerful metaphor on change for overloaded child protection systems (TSA 2007). Following the September 11th terrorist aircraft attacks and the Richard Reid shoe bomb attempt in 2001, the TSA banned cigarette lighters in carry-on luggage. As of August 4, 2007 the TSA reversed this decision explaining:

> Lifting the lighter ban is consistent with TSA's risk-based approach to aviation security. First and foremost, lighters no longer pose a significant threat. Freeing security officers up from fishing for 22,000 lighters every day (the current number surrendered daily across the country) enables them to focus more on finding explosives, using behavior recognition, conducting random screening procedures and other measures that increase complexity in the system, deterring terrorists.
>
> (TSA 2007: web page 1)

In essence, the TSA reversed its cigarette lighter ban because it was counterproductive to the real issue at hand—detecting and preventing terrorist attacks on airlines—and it misused valuable time and human resources. The problem was that in focusing on minor risks, the more serious risks would be missed. Returning to child protection, we can see similarities between it and the previous approach of the TSA. Reasons such as using ever-wider definitions of harm and trawling through copious amounts of mostly insignificant reports in search of those allegations that involve serious risk to vulnerable children are in fact counterproductive to the overall aim of protecting children and enhancing their safety and well-being. Moreover, scarce resources are diverted on unnecessary and intrusive investigations, rather than providing real help to those in need. Like the TSA, child protection advocates need to have the courage to face up to the evidence and the array of indicators which show that current protective policies and structures are not working and are unworkable, to the point where they threaten the sustainability of the overall protective systems for vulnerable children and families.

In addition, we argue for a re-emphasis of civil society rather than just systemic reform of child protection. Our focus on child and family well-being aims to realign the relations between the state and families in order to provide social care to those who are vulnerable and in need. Continuing with overly harsh, punitive, and intrusive processes will only further marginalize those groups who are already significantly excluded from Anglophone societies.

Our proposals entail a significant realignment of the social care and social control mandates in order to ensure that the system overall, and the specific interventions into family life, have a broader base than just safety by also having enhanced child and family well-being as central features. This means rethinking the language of child protection such as "harm," "abuse," and "safety" is required, along with a commitment to broader understandings of what is in children's (and families') best interests in both the short and longer terms.

Reshaping the practitioner–service user relations to ensure that there is a strong guiding value base underpinning the social care that is provided will significantly reorient services, as well as positively alter the outcomes for children and families. More than ever, we need a strong evidence base to ascertain the success or otherwise of these social interventions, and to guide the necessary reforms. Clear guiding principles are that protective and other interventions must have justice and positive outcomes for all parties as imperatives to policy formulation and practice. For example, it is simply unacceptable to have the life outcomes of children in care being so poor in comparison to other children. A reformed child protection system will see "care alumni" as having high-order needs that require enhanced support and assistance rather than judgmental risk-driven assessments that further marginalize and ostracize. Positive life outcomes for those who have been the most seriously abused and neglected and required protective removal does not, in our view, seem unattainable or too costly. Quite the opposite, trans-generational trauma as a consequence for those who have not been able to be cared for by their families is morally unacceptable and leads to high service costs.

Our guiding principles include having a child-centered, family-focused and culturally respectful framework for interventions. For Indigenous children and families, in particular, this is imperative. Current systems continue to live with the legacy of earlier policies that had far-reaching negative consequences for generations of Indigenous peoples, with trauma and a host of social, health, and economic consequences continuing to plague these communities. Yet, despite the overwhelming evidence of the deplorable situation for many Indigenous communities, governments are often reluctant to either provide the necessary resources or the policy frameworks that promote self-determination and economic self-sufficiency. Socially just child and family well-being programs have an important part to play in helping disadvantaged and marginalized Indigenous people to address the trans-generational trauma, provide necessary support and practical assistance to redress the chronic needs, and attend to the economic exclusion.

There are, of course, other groups of people who have tended to be squarely in the sights of child protection authorities and who also have high-order needs, such as people who are poor, have mental illness or disability, single parents (particularly women), people of color, and those who are socially excluded. Effective child and family well-being systems also need to attend to broader issues rather than just focusing on safety for the vulnerable. Our restructured service delivery system is better able to render this broad-based assistance to unmet social and economic need, and thereby prevent many of the family issues that are currently left to fester until they become serious enough to warrant child protection responses.

The voices, concerns and aspirations of those most directly affected by protective and other social care interventions must have opportunities for being heard in a reformed system. We have called for a reinvigorated approach to partnership that places service users central to the decision-making processes in both policy formulation and service implementation. At present, children in particular remain largely on the periphery, although there are notable examples where innovative approaches are responding directly to their needs. Practitioners and managers in a robust child and family well-being system will draw upon their practical wisdom in listening to and incorporating service user perspectives to inform and guide their practice and policies. Child- and family-friendly systems are characterized by clear and accessible pathways for help and support, with services embedded within neighborhoods and communities. We have proposed a number of structural initiatives that will facilitate community involvement and participation into service delivery systems so that the voices of services users and stakeholders are given rightful spaces to be heard. Community members, child advocates, educators, professional associations, the media, and politicians are allies in the reform process and change agendas.

In our proposed child and family well-being system, relationship-based practice is a hallmark of social care interventions and practice. We feel strongly that change at the individual and family systems levels is to a large extent dependent upon the abilities of practitioners to inspire people to aspire. Using themselves as facilitators of change, skilled and effective social workers and human service practitioners use their relationships as a process for people to explore their issues, perspectives on life, and others, and to encourage them to commit to changing their lives and turning things around. The potential power for personal change, growth and development in traumatized and damaged people that practitioners can bring to bear is awe inspiring, and an invaluable tool for enhancing safety and well-being in vulnerable and troubled people. We have also noted that with this sort of powerful ability, it is essential for practitioners to engage in reflective practice so that they are fully cognizant of the relationships and psychodynamic processes that are taking place and the ethical and other issues at play. Traumatized people can be very needy and vulnerable and highly ethical practitioners are aware of this and of the boundaries around sound practice approaches.

An ethical framework

It is lamentable that contemporary child protection, which typically entails working with very vulnerable people in situations where power and authority imbalances characterize the relationships and contact, does not have a clearly articulated framework for ethical practice. Our book has gone some way toward developing this but more work is needed to flesh out these principles and processes so that practitioners can ensure that they practice in a fit and proper way, cognizant of their moral and other obligations. At present, practitioners are usually left to depend on organizational or disciplinary-based codes, which are useful, but fall well short of ensuring ethics are embodied in their everyday practice.

Child protection and child and family well-being practice is, however, quintessentially moral work that goes to issues including justice, social justice, power, caring, authority, and vulnerability. In Chapter 8 we articulated a virtue ethics framework that focuses on three conceptual elements: competing ethical principles, unequal power relationships, and complex stakeholder responsibilities. Virtue ethics utilizes an approach that bridges ethical principles and the outcomes of our actions, so that in child protection we do not just adhere to an ethical code but consider closely what the likely outcomes might be and then make a decision about the best course of action in accordance with a person of integrity—or as Tobin (1994: 55) notes, someone who can be trusted to act in a fit and proper way. Meagher and Parton (2004) outlined how practice characterized by an ethic of care would look, and this is in accord with the tenets of virtue ethics.

Essentially, a virtue ethics approach to child and family well-being requires practitioners to adopt the notion of being a moral agent in carrying out their duties, mindful of relevant ethical principles (such as best interests, do no harm, justice) and to also incorporate into their decision making considerations of the possible outcomes for those affected. This ethical framework does not ignore or shy away from the complex and vexed issues in determining proper conduct. Rather, it directly confronts these and places a responsibility on the practitioner to be able to clearly articulate and justify the ethical rationale for their decision making and actions. It expects professionals making these difficult determinations to be familiar with competing ethical principles, comprehend the power dynamics at play in their multiple relationships, and to understand their duties and obligations to all those stakeholders who have an interest in a matter, particularly the child and parents.

In advocating a virtue ethics approach for child and family well-being practitioners we also challenge the narrow and sometime exclusive use of the "best interests of the child" principle, which is embedded in nearly all legislative and policy frameworks in Anglophone countries. Without an appreciation of the fact that applying the "best interest" principle offers nothing more than a focus for assessment, it risks being used as template for action where decisions are defended without any justification other than "this is in the best interests." On what basis is this defended? The best interest for the present or the future? And most importantly, whose perspective of "best interest" is used? Or excluded? When combined with the risk-averse and power-laden organizational cultures that typify many child protection agencies, this principle is often used singularly as the only ethical principle relevant to protective decision making. We believe that, just as risk assessment tools usually require short-term time frames for decision making, such approaches are often at odds with other ethical principles that incorporate broader notions of best practice, and more appropriate time frames in determining the consequences of decision making and protective inter-ventions. In short, at present, practitioners are encouraged to look no further than the immediate situation in making decisions. This has had profound implications for the lives and life outcomes of service users, and, ultimately, the broader community.

We have proposed that best practice is for child protection and child and family well-being practice to have ethical practice at its core—driving the decision making and interventions with the overarching goal being to build a better, robust, and caring civil society. Practitioners should be knowledgeable of, and comfortable with, a range of competing ethical principles so that they can apply these with judicious wisdom into situations that are inherently complex, challenging and uncertain. Knowing their legal responsibilities including duty of care and how these also shape practice is essential. Furthermore, given the pivotal part that relationship plays, practitioners need to be conversant with the fluid dynamics that power differentials play in the social care and social control aspects of their work, reflect on these, and use their authority in ways that empower and build the capacity of service users, particularly children. Finally, effective child and family well-being practitioners understand and take into account their ethical duties to a range of other stakeholders in the broader family, neighborhood, and community who have an interest in the care of children and families and the systems established to enhance their well-being. Awareness of their duties and obligations will assist them in being able to clearly articulate and justify the reasons for their decisions and actions on behalf of the broad community.

Organizational and service delivery models

Our proposals for altered organizational and service delivery models emerge from critical analysis and careful consideration of the dynamic factors shaping organizational and service user outcomes, the range of reform initiatives previously undertaken, and the readily evident ongoing problems affecting service users, staff, and other stakeholders. Of particular note is the large list of previously attempted changes to policy and practice that have usually resulted in further failures. We concluded that important initiatives such as differential response have largely been unsuccessful because the reform process was usually akin to minor modifications that do not properly address the fundamental problems. For example, differential response policies can also be held accountable for any systemic failures, such as when a child dies. Therefore, more wide-sweeping reforms are needed lest further failure results from a narrow change agenda.

We appreciate that people may well baulk at the scope and scale of our proposals and chart different courses. We are not suggesting that all our proposals should be implemented without serious analysis of the local context and issues. Explicit in the framework we propose is the centrality of culture, relationship, and location in determining "best practice" rather than universal protocols or procedures. Much time, energy and resources are spent on organizational restructuring, with failure often being the result if there is also no attendant focus on the legislative, policy, ethical, and practice frameworks so that practitioners can operate in the ways we have suggested. We have tried to encompass all these domains within a comprehensive agenda that will change the underlying value-base to the social relations upon which social care and social control responses are based. Altered structures will probably not work unless there are other simultaneous changes. However, we remain confident that an overwhelming proportion of practitioners, service users, and stakeholders from the broad community in Anglophone countries recognize the unworkability and unsustainability of current approaches. People are ready for reform as long as they can be convinced that, like our proposals, it addresses the issues at hand and will lead to better outcomes.

Identifying the distinct roles and functions of a comprehensive child and family well-being system and then splitting the responsibilities and accountabilities into separate organizational entities we believe makes the overall social mandate and organizational missions clearer and more likely to be achieved. While super departments may be more administratively efficient (although this is debatable), we posit that their complexity and multi-mission tasks render them incapable of being effective service deliverers, and therefore unlikely to achieve positive outcomes for service users, particularly children in care, and the community. While the rhetorical justifications for putting the competing functions of social control and social care into the same organizations include greater programatic integration, better communication and improved coordination of service delivery, we would argue that there is little hard evidence to demonstrate the success of this approach. Organizations that have clear social mandates and missions are far more likely to be successful in meeting their objectives because they can remain focused on "core business," without the often unrealistic community expectations that they must be all things to all people. Moreover, separate organizations means that there is less chance of child protection investigative functions squeezing out the equally important (some might say more important) helping preventative requirements. Service users are tired of being vilified and punished, but not being given the help they desperately need when they ask for it.

We suggest that an important role of Community Child and Family Well-being Boards will be to make these structures and intervention processes keep the right balance between social care and social control, and between primary and secondary prevention, and tertiary interventions. Besides providing a key and influential forum for the voice of service users and community stakeholders, they provide a check and balance to ensure that policy and practice is in accord with broad community standards and expectations. They will help to keep these organizations truly accountable but not in ways that are merely punitive and blaming. Regular review and evaluations will take place under their gaze. Furthermore, these Boards will be able to advocate for a robust role and involvement for the community-based not-for-profit and for-profit agencies and practitioners so that community members can access the sorts of services and assistance that they require to meet their needs. To be an effective system, it is critical for the community-based non-government organizations to play a full and proper part within a fully integrated structure of social care, particularly for those who are marginalized and socially excluded.

Our child and family well-being system is built on the principles of a public health model, which recognizes and does not shirk from risk, nor sets hopelessly unrealistic expectations that no child will be harmed or killed. Rather, the system emphasizes reducing the rates of abuse and neglect victimization through a range of preventative programs and measures, at the primary, secondary, and tertiary levels. The system also has an orientation toward holistic and longer term assistance, rather than narrower interventions that have unrealistic timeframes for individual and family changes to be effected. Moreover, because principles and processes for facilitating restorative justice are incorporated into our system proposals, there are more likely to be proper responses to the damage that occurs to interpersonal relationships when abuse and neglect occurs.

Importantly, our proposed systems do not reject NPM outright because we recognize that the emphasis on sound strategic and operational planning is essential when undertaking significant organizational changes, as are the utilization of a range of business practices that can improve the focus on service user outcomes. We do, however, assert that NPM has significant shortcomings, particularly insofar as it reshapes organizational power relations at a variety of levels, and is dominated by a managerial discourse to the significant detriment of professional practice and service user outcomes. We are convinced that human service organizations that embrace practice-informed approaches to management are far more likely to be effective in reaching their organizational mission and objectives. Effective human service organizations have strong, capable, and engaged management and skilled, knowledgeable, and reflective front-line staff, with all employees conversant with the organizational mission and the methods for achieving desired goals and objectives.

Crisis? What crisis?

We have outlined an array of evidence to demonstrate that, despite considerable achievements in protecting children and families, contemporary approaches to child protection in Anglophone counties are seriously flawed and often counterproductive, and that these child protection systems are failing and unsustainable in their present configurations. Further, the demonstrable outcomes for the range of service users and key stakeholders are not in accord-ance with the social mandate for these systems, and are contrary to the aspirations of civil society, which adheres to principles of social justice, fairness and compassion, and care and protection for the vulnerable. We have presented a fully justified and compelling case for reform. Nevertheless, some people might read this book and dispute the seriousness of the problems for child protection systems that we have detailed. They may say "Crisis? What crisis?" While we understand that the situation is not as dire as we portray in all jurisdictions, we nevertheless reject arguments that suggest tinker-ing modifications to child protection systems are sufficient to remedy the problems. More of the same way, with little-by-little changes, will not address the iatrogenesis that characterizes current Anglophone approaches to child protection, which are demonstrating terrible consequences for the lives of many vulnerable children, parents and families—problems that are trans-generational.

Fundamental reform processes take time to implement and bed down, and we have outlined processes and mechanisms for achieving successful change management. We remain confident that reforms such as we have outlined will provide a solid foundation for improving the lot of people who come into contact with child protection systems. At the very least, we hope that we have provided much food for thought and advanced the debates that the broad community and human services sectors must have if we are to address the problems that beset our current systems of protection and alternative care for children who are not able to reside at home. We are confident that there is the collective will to provide for children, parents, and families in Anglophone civil societies, the safety, security, and enhanced well-being that a morally engaged late modern society based on justice and fairness for all is able to provide. Positive outcomes for service users and the broad community are requisite results for child and family well-being systems and services. The general public expects no less. Children, parents and families requiring help deserve no less. Reforming child protection is timely and, perhaps more importantly, is the right thing to do.

References

ABC News (2007) "Aboriginal Infants Returned to Families," Wed. December 5. Online. Available www.abc.net.au/news/stories/2007/12/05/2109828.htm?section= justin (accessed December 7, 2007).

Abramovitz, M. (2005) "The largely untold story of welfare reform and the human services," *Social Work*, 50(2): 175–86.

Adams, P. and Chandler, S. (2004) "Responsive regulation in child welfare: Systemic challenges in mainstreaming the family group conference," *Journal of Sociology and Social Welfare*, 31(1): 93–116.

AIHW (2006) *Child Protection Australia 2005–06*, Canberra: Australian Institute of Health and Welfare.

Ainsworth, F. (2002) "Mandatory reporting of child abuse and neglect: does it really make a difference?" *Child and Family Social Work*, 7(1): 57–64.

Ainsworth, F. and Hansen, P. (2006) "Five tumultuous years in Australian child protection: Little progress," *Child and Family Social Work*, 11(1): 33–41.

Aldgate, J. (2002) "Evolution not revolution: Family support services and the Children Act 1989," in H. Ward and W. Rose (eds) *Approaches to Needs Assessment in Children's Services*, London: Jessica Kingsley.

Anderson, D. (2000) "Coping strategies and burnout among veteran child protection workers," *Child Abuse and Neglect*, 24(6): 839–48.

Anderson, M. and Gobeil, S. (2002) *Recruitment and Retention in Child Welfare Services: A Survey of Child Welfare League of Canada Member Agencies*, Ottawa, Ontario: Center of Excellence for Child Welfare, Child Welfare League of Canada.

Anheier, H. (ed.) (1999) *When Things Go Wrong: Organizational Failures and Breakdowns*, London: Sage Publications.

Archard, D. (1993) *Children: Rights and Childhood*, London: Routledge.

Argy, F. (2004) "Balancing conflicting goals: The big challenge for government," *Australian Journal of Public Administration*, 63(4): 22–8.

Aronson, J. and Sammon, S. (2000) "Practice amid social service restructuring: Working with the contradictions of 'small victories'," *Canadian Social Work Review*, 17(2): 167–87.

Ashenden, S. (1996) "Reflective governance and child sexual abuse: Liberal welfare rationality and the Cleveland Inquiry," *Economy and Society*, 24(1): 64–88.

—— (2004) *Governing Child Sexual Abuse: Negotiating the Boundaries of Public and Private, Law and Science*, London: Routledge.

Ashford, J. (2006) "Comparing the effects of judicial versus child protective relationships on parental attitudes in the juvenile dependency process," *Research on Social Work Practice*, 16(6): 582–90.

Asquith, M. and Cheers, B. (2001) "Morals, ethics and practice: In search of social justice," *Australian Social Work*, 54(2): 15–26.

Audit Commission (1994) *Seen But Not Heard: Coordinating Community Health and Social Services for Children in Need*, London: HMSO.

Australian Senate Community Affairs References Committee (2001a) *Lost Innocents: Righting the Record*, Canberra: Australian Government Printing Service.

—— (2001b) *Forgotten Australians: A Report on Australians who Experienced Institutional Out-of-home Care as Children*, Canberra: Australian Government Printing Service.

—— (2005) *Protecting Vulnerable Children: A National Challenge, Second Report on the Inquiry into Children in Institutional Care*, Canberra: Senate Printing Unit, Parliament House.

Bakwin, H. (1956) "Multiple skeletal lesions in young children due to trauma," *Pediatrics*, 49: 7–15.

Banks, S. (2006) *Ethics and Values in Social Work*, 3rd edn, London: Palgrave.

Barter, K. (2002) "Enough is enough: Renegotiating relationships to create a conceptual revolution in community and children's protection," *Canada's Children*, Ottawa: Child Welfare League of Canada.

Barton, A. and Welbourne, P. (2005) "Context and its significance in identifying 'What Works' in child protection," *Child Abuse Review*, 14: 177–94.

Bath, H. (2000) "Rights and realities in the permanency debate," *Children Australia*, 25(4): 13–17.

Bauman, Z. (1993) *Postmodern Ethics*, London: Polity Press.

Bean, P. and Melville J. (1989) *Lost Children of the Empire*, London: Unwin Hyman.

Beauchamp, T. and Childress, J. (2001) *Principles of Biomedical Ethics*, 5th edn, New York: Oxford University Press.

Beck, U. and Beck-Gernsheim, E. (2002) *Individualization: Institutionalized Individualism and its Social and Political Consequences*, London: Sage.

Beckett, C. and Maynard, A. (2005) *Values & Ethics in Social Work*, London: Sage Publications.

Bednar, S.G. (2003) "Elements satisfying organisational climates in child welfare agencies," *Families in Society*, 84(1): 7–12.

Behlmer, G.K. (1982) *Child Abuse and Moral Reform in England, 1870–1908*, Stanford, CA: Stanford University Press.

Bell, S. (1988) *When Salem Came to the Boro: The True Story of the Cleveland Child Abuse Crisis*, London: Pan Books.

Bellefeuille, G. and Schmidt, G. (2006) "Between a rock and a hard place: Child welfare practice and social work education," *Social Work Education*, 25(1): 3–16.

Beresford, P. and Croft, S. (1980) *Community Control of Social Services Departments*, London: Battersea Community Action.

—— and —— (1993) *Citizen Involvement: A Practical Guide for Change*, London: Macmillan.

—— and —— (2004) "Service users and practitioners reunited: The key component for social work reform," *British Journal of Social Work*, 34: 53–68.

Berg, I.K. and Kelly, S. (2000) *Building Solutions in Child Protective Services*, New York: W.W. Norton & Co.

Berridge, D. (2007) "Theory and explanation in child welfare: Education and looked after children," *Child and Family Social Work*, 12: 1–10.

Berry, M. (1997) *The Family at Risk: Issues and Trends in Family Preservation Services*, Columbia: University of South Carolina Press.

Besharov, D. (1988) "The need to narrow the grounds for state intervention", in D. Besharov (ed.) *Protecting Children from Abuse and Neglect: Policy and Practice*, Springfield, IL: C.C. Thomas.

—— (1990) "Gaining control over child abuse reports: Public agencies must address both underreporting and overreporting," *Public Welfare*, 48: 34–40.

Blaskett, B. and Taylor, S.C. (2003) *Facilitators and Inhibitors of Mandatory Reporting of Suspected Child Abuse*, Canberra: Australian Institute of Criminology. Online. Available www.aic.gov.au/crc/reports/200102-09.pdf (accessed October 1, 2007).

Blewett, J., Lewis. J. and Tunstill, J. (2007) *The Changing Roles and Tasks of Social Work: A Literature Informed Discussion Paper*, London: General Social Care Council.

Boateng, P. (1999) "The Government's role in early intervention" (speech to a conference on the importance of early intervention held in London, March 12, 1998), in R. Bayley (ed.) *Transforming Children's Lives: The Importance of Early Intervention. Occasional Paper 25*, London: Family Policy Studies Center.

Bradley, L. and Parker, R. (2006) "Do Australian public sector employees have the type of culture they want in the era of new public management?" *Australian Journal of Public Administration*, 65(1): 89–99.

Braithwaite, J. (2004) "Families and the Republic," *Journal of Sociology and Social Welfare*, 31(1): 199–215.

Brandon, M., Thoburn, J., Lewis, A. and Wade, J. (1999) *Safeguarding Children with the Children Act 1989*, London: Stationery Office.

Bridgman, P. and Davis, G. (2004) *The Australian Policy Handbook*, 3rd edn, Sydney: Allen and Unwin.

Brodkin, E.Z. (2000) *Investigating Policy's "Practical" Meaning: Street level research on welfare policy*, Chicago: Joint Center for Poverty Research, North Western University/University of Chicago. Online. Available www.jcpr.org/wp/Wpprofile.dfm?ID=169 (accessed October 6, 2007).

Bromfield, L. and Higgins, D. (2005) "National comparisons of Child Protection Systems," *Child Abuse Prevention Issues*, Melbourne: National Child Protection Clearing House—Australian Institute of Family Studies. Online. Available www.aifs.gov.au/nch/pubs/issues/issues22/issues22.html#author (accessed December 3, 2007).

Brown, J.D. and Bednar, L.M. (2006) "Foster Parent Perceptions of Placement Breakdown," *Children and Youth Services Review*, 28: 1497–1511.

Buckley, H. (2003) *Child Protection Work: Beyond the Rhetoric*, London: Jessica Kingsley Publishers.

Butcher, A. (2005) "Upping the ante!; The training and status of foster carers in Queensland", *Children Australia*, 30(3): 25–30.

Buti, A. (2002) "British Child Migration to Australia: History, Senate Inquiry and Responsibilities", *Murdoch University Electronic Journal of Law*, 9(4). Online. Available www.murdoch.edu.au/elaw/issues/v9n4/buti94.html (accessed August 18, 2007).

Burford, G. and Adams, P. (2004) "Restorative justice, responsive regulation and social work," *Journal of Sociology and Social Welfare*, 31(1): 7–26.

Butler, I. and Drakeford, M. (2005) *Scandal, Social Policy and Social Welfare*, Bristol: Policy Press.

Caffey, J. (1946) "Multiple fractures in the long bones of infants suffering from chronic subdural hematoma," *American Journal of Roentgenology*, 56: 1008–14.

Callahan, M. (2000) "Valuing the Field: Lessons from Innovation", in M. Callahan, S. Hessle and S. Strega, S. (eds) *Valuing the Field: Child Welfare in an International Context*. Aldershot: Ashgate.

Cheers, B., Darracott, R. and Lonne, B. (2007) *Social Care Practice in Rural Communities*, Annandale NSW: Federation Press.

Chevannes, M. (2002) "Social construction of the managerialism of needs assessment by health and social care professionals," *Health and Social Care in the Community* 10(3): 168–78.

Chief Secretary to the Treasury (2003) *Every Child Matters* (Cm 5860), London: Stationery Office.

Child Welfare Information Gateway (2006) *Child Abuse and Neglect Fatalities: Statistics and interventions*, Washington, DC: US Department of Health and Human Services.

Churchill, W. (1994) *Indians Are Us?: Culture and Genocide in Native North America*, Maine, USA: Common Courage Books.

Clark, C. (2000) *Social Work Ethics: Politics, Principles and Practice*, Hampshire: Macmillan Press.

Cohen, S. (2002) *Folk Devils and Moral Panics: The Creation of the Mods and the Rockers*, 3rd edn, London. Routledge.

Congress, E. and McAuliffe, D. (2006) "Social work ethics: Professional codes in Australia and the United States," *International Social Work*, 49: 151–64.

Connolly, M. and Doolan, M. (2006) "Child deaths and statutory services: Issues for child care and protection," *Communities, Families and Children Australia*, 2(1): 26–37.

—— and —— (2007) "Responding to the deaths of children known to child protection agencies," *Social Policy Journal of New Zealand*, 30: 1–11.

Cooper, A. (2002) "International Perspectives in Child Protection," in M. Hill, A. Stafford and P. Green Lister (eds) *International Perspectives on Child Protection: Report of a Seminar Held on 20 March 2002*. Glasgow: University of Glasgow.

——, Hetherington, R., Bairstow, K., Pitts, J. and Spriggs, A. (1995) *Positive Child Protection: A View from Abroad*, Lyme Regis: Russell House Publishing.

——, —— and Katz, I. (2003) *The Risk Factor: Making the Child Protection System Work*, London: Demos. Online. Available www.demos.co.uk/publications/riskfactor (accessed March 23, 2007).

Cooper, L. (2002) "Social work supervision: A social justice perspective", in M. McMahon and W. Patton (eds) *Supervision in the Helping Professions: A Practical Approach*, Sydney: Pearson Education Australia.

Corby, B., Doig, A. and Roberts, V. (1998) "Inquiries into Child Abuse," *Journal of Social Welfare and Family Law*, 20(4): 377–95.

Courtney, M. and Dworsky, A. (2006) "Early outcomes for young adults transitioning from out-of-home care in the USA," *Child & Family Social Work*, 11: 209–19.

Crampton, D. (2004) "Family involvement interventions in child protection: Learning from contextual integration strategies," *Journal of Sociology and Social Welfare*, 31(1): 175–98.

Crime and Misconduct Commission (CMC) (2004) *Protecting Children: An Inquiry into Abuse of Children in Foster Care*, Brisbane: Crime and Misconduct Commission.

Cunneen, C. and Libesman, T. (2000) "Postcolonial Trauma: The contemporary removal of Indigneous children and young people from their families in Australia," *Australian Journal of Social Issues*, 35(2): 99–115.

Dale, P. (2004) "'Like a fish in a bowl': Parents perceptions of child protection services," *Child Abuse Review*, 13: 137–57.

Daro, D., Budd, S., Baker, S., Nesmith, A. and Harden, A. (2005) *Community Partnerships for Protecting Children: Phase II Outcome Evaluation, Final Report*, Chicago, IL: Chapin Hall Center for Children.

Darwall, S. (ed.) (2003) *Virtue Ethics*, Malden, MA: Blackwell Publishing.

Dawson, K. and Berry, M. (2002) "Engaging families in child welfare services: An evidence-based approach to best practice," *Child Welfare*, 81(2): 293–318.

de Boer, C. and Coady, N. (2007) "Good helping relationships in child welfare: Learning from stories of success," *Child and Family Social Work*, 12: 32–42.

Department of Child Safety (2006) "Peer and employee support service wins Premier's award," Brisbane, Queensland, Department of Child Safety. Online. Available www.childsafety.qld.gov.au/magazine/2007-01/features1.html (accessed October 9, 2007).

Department for Education and Skills (2004) *Every Child Matters: Next Steps*, London: Stationery Office.

Department of Family and Children's Services (1996) *New Directions in Child Protection and Family Support—Interim Guidelines, Standards and Implementation Package*, Perth: Department of Family and Children's Services.

Department of Health (1995) *Child Protection: Messages from Research*, London: HMSO.

—— (2001) *The Children Act Now: Messages from Research*, London: Stationery Office.

Department of Health, Department of Education and Employment, Home Office (2000) *Framework for the Assessment of Children in Need and their Families*, London: Stationery Office.

Department of Health, Home Office, Department of Education and Employment (1999) *Working Together to Safeguard Children: A Guide to Inter-Agency Working to Safeguard and Promote the Welfare of Children*, London: Stationery Office.

DHSS (1982) *Child Abuse: A Study of Inquiry Reports 1973–1981*, London: HMSO.

Diefenbach, T. (2007) "The managerialistic ideology of organisational change management," *Journal of Organizational Change Management*, 20(1): 126–44.

Dingwall, R. (1989) "Some Problems about Predicting Child Abuse and Neglect," in O. Stevenson (ed.) *Child Abuse: Public Policy and Professional Practice*, Hemel Hempstead: Harvester Wheatsheaf.

Dingwall, R., Eekelaar, J. and Murray, T. (1995) "Postscript," *The Protection of Children: State Intervention and Family Life*, 2nd edn, Oxford: Basil Blackwell.

Doka, K.J. (1989) *Disenfranchised Grief: Recognising Hidden Sorrow*, Lexington: Lexington Books.

Dollard, M., Winefield, H.R. and Winefield, A.H. (2001) *Occupational Strain and Efficacy in Human Service Workers: When the Rescuer Becomes the Victim*, London: Kluwer Academic Publishers.

Dumbrill, G. (2003) "Child welfare: AOP's nemesis?" in W. Shera (ed.) *Emerging Perspectives on Anti-Oppressive Practice*, Toronto: Canadian Scholars' Press.

—— (2006) "Parental experience of child protection intervention: A qualitative study," *Child Abuse and Neglect*, 30: 27–37.

Dunifon, R., Hynes, K. and Peters, H. (2006) "Welfare reform and child well-being," *Children and Youth Services Review*, 28: 1273–92.

Ellett, A., Ellis, J., Westbrook, T. and Dews, D. (2007) "A qualitative study of 369 child welfare professionals perspectives about factors contributing to employee retention and turnover," *Children and Youth Services Review*, 29: 264–81.

Ellis, G. (2000) "Reflective learning and supervision," in L. Cooper and L. Briggs (eds) *Fieldwork in the Human Services: Theory and Practice for Field Educators, Practice Teachers and Supervisors*, Sydney: Allen and Unwin.

English, D., Wingard, T., Marshall, D., Orme, M. and Orme, A. (2000) "Alternative responses to child protective services," *Child Abuse and Neglect*, 24(3): 378–88.

Evans, T. and Harris, J. (2006) "A case of mistaken identity? Debating the dilemmas of street-level bureaucracy with Musil *et al.*," *European Journal of Social Work*, 9(4): 445–59.

Family Inclusion Network (2007) *Family Inclusion in Child Protection Practice: Supporting Families, Stronger Futures*, Queensland: Family Inclusion Network.

Farell, A. (2004) "Child protection policy perspectives and reform of Australian legislation," *Child Abuse Review*, 13: 234–45.

Fawcett, B., Featherstone, B. and Goddard, J. (2004) *Contemporary Child Care Policy and Practice*, Basingstoke: Palgrave Macmillan.

Featherstone, B. (2004) *Family Life and Family Support: A Feminist Analysis*, Basingstoke: Palgrave Macmillan.

—— (2006) "Rethinking family support in the current policy context," *British Journal of Social Work*, 36(1): 5–20.

Ferguson, H. (1990) "Rethinking child protection practices: A case for history," in The Violence Against Children Study Group *Taking Child Abuse Seriously*, London: Unwin Hyman.

—— (1996) "The protection of children in time," *Child and Family Social Work*, 1(4): 205–18.

—— (1997) "Protecting children in new times: Child protection and the risk society," *Child and Family Social Work*, 2(4): 221–34.

—— (2004) *Protecting Children in Time: Child Abuse, Child Protection and the Consequences of Modernity*, Basingstoke: Palgrave Macmillan.

Finkelhor, D. (1990) "Is child abuse overreported?" *Public Welfare*, 46(1): 22–9.

—— and L. Jones (2006) "Why have child maltreatment and child victimization declined?" *Journal of Social Issues*, 62(4): 685–716.

Fisher, T., Gibbs, I., Sinclair, I. and Wilson, K. (2000) "Sharing the care: the qualities sought of social workers by foster carers," *Child and Family Social Work*, 5: 225–33.

Fook, J. (2004) "Critical reflection and transformative possibilities," in L. Davies and P. Leonard (eds) *Social Work in a Corporate Era: Practices of Power and Resistance*. Burlington, VT.: Ashgate.

Ford, P. (2007) *Review of the Department for Community Development; Review Report*, Perth, Western Australia: Government of Western Australia.

Fournier, S. and Crey, E. (1997) *Stolen from our Embrace: The Abduction of First Nations Children and the Restoration of Aboriginal Communities*, Vancouver: Douglas and McIntyre.

Fox Harding, L. (1996) *Family, State & Social Policy*, Basingstoke: Macmillan.

France, A. and Utting, D. (2005) "The paradigm of 'risk and protection-focused prevention' and its impact on services for children and families," *Children & Society*, 19(2): 77–90.

Franklin, B. (1989) "Wimps and Bullies: Press Reporting of Child Abuse," in P. Carter, T. Jeffs and M. Smith (eds) *Social Work and Social Welfare Yearbook One*, Buckingham: Open University Press.

Freymond, N. (2003) *Mother's Everyday Realities and Child Placement Experiences*, Partnerships for Children and Families Project. Online. Available www.wlu.ca/docsnpubs_detail.php?grp_id=1288&doc_id=7217 (accessed December 10, 2007).

—— and Cameron, G. (2006) (eds) *Toward Positive Systems of Child and Family Welfare*, Toronto: University of Toronto Press.

Friedman, M. (1958) "Traumatic periostitis in infants and children," *Journal of American Medical Association*, 2: 1840–5.

Froggett, L. (2002) *Love, Hate and Welfare: Psychosocial Approaches to Policy and Practice*, Bristol: The Policy Press.

Gambrill, E. and Shlonsky, A. (2001) "The need for comprehensive risk management systems in child welfare," *Children and Youth Services Review*, 23(1): 79–107.

Gibbons, J., Conroy, S. and Bell, C. (1995) *Operating the Child Protection System*, London: HMSO.

Giddens, A. (1990) *The Consequences of Modernity*, Cambridge: Polity Press.

Gilbert, N. (ed.) (1997) *Combating Child Abuse: International Perspectives and Trends*, Oxford: Oxford University Press.

—— (2002) *Transformation of the Welfare State: The Silent Surrender of Public Responsibility*, New York: Oxford University Press.

Gilbertson, R. and Barber, J.G. (2003) "Breakdown of foster care placement: carer perspectives and system factors," *Australian Social Work*, 56(4): 329–39.

—— and —— (2004) "The systemic abrogation of practice standards in foster care," *Australian Social Work*, 57(1): 31–45.

Gilligan, C. (1982) *In a Different Voice: Psychological Theory and Women's Development*, Cambridge, MA: Harvard University Press.

Glisson, C., Dukes, D., and Green, P. (2006) "The effects of ARC organizational intervention on caseworker turnover, climate, and culture in children's services systems," *Child Abuse and Neglect*, 30: 855–80.

—— and Hemmelgarn, A. (1998) "The effects of organizational climate and inter-organizational coordination on the quality and outcomes of children's service systems," *Child Abuse and Neglect*, 22(5): 401–21.

Gordon, L. (1989) *Heroes of Their Own Lives: The Politics and History of Family Violence*, London: Virago.

Gray, J. (2002) "National Policy on the Assessment of Children in Need and their Families," in H. Ward and W. Rose (eds) *Approaches to Needs Assessment in Children's Services*, London: Jessica Kingsley.

Gray, M. and Gibbons, J. (2007) "There are no answers, only choices: Teaching ethical decision making in social work," *Australian Social Work*, 60(2): 222–38.

Gupta, A. and Blewett, J. (2007) "Change for children? The challenges and opportunities for the children's social work workforce," *Child and Family Social Work*, 12: 172–81.

Hacking, I. (1988) "The Sociology of Knowledge about Child Abuse," *Nous*, 2: 53–63.

—— (1991) "The making and moulding of child abuse," *Critical Inquiry*, 17 (Winter): 253–88.

—— (1992) "World-making by kind-making: Child abuse for example," in M. Douglas and D. Hull (eds) *How Classification Works: Nelson Goodman among the Social Sciences*, Edinburgh: Edinburgh University Press.

Halpern, R. (1991) "Supportive services to families in poverty: Dilemma of reform," *Social Services Review*, 65: 343–64.

Hanlon, A. (1966) "From social reform to social security: The separation of ADC and child welfare," *Child Welfare*, 45: 109–20.

Hansen, P. and Ainsworth, F. (under review) "From prevention to punishment: Developments in child protection in New South Wales."

Harder, M.H. and Pringle, K. (eds) (1997) *Protecting Children in Europe: Toward a New Millennium*, Aalborg: Aalborg University Press.

Hardy, M., Schibler, B. and Hamilton, I. (2006) *Strengthen the Commitment: An External Review of the Child Welfare System*, Manitoba: Report commissioned by Minister of Family Services and Housing.

Harries, M. and Clare, M. (2002) *Mandatory Reporting of Child Abuse: Evidence and Options*, Perth, Western Australia: Discipline of Social Work & Social Policy, University of Western Australia.

——, Harris, P., Diamond, S. and Mackenzie, G. (2004) *Caring Well—Protecting Well: investing in systemic responses to protect children in WA*, Report for The Ministerial Advisory Council on Child Protection Western Australia, Perth, Western Australia: The Ministerial Advisory Council on Child Protection Western Australia.

Harris, J. (1998) "Scientific management, bureau-professionalism, New managerialism: The labor process of state social work," *British Journal of Social Work*, 28: 839–62.

Hart, M.A. (2002) *Seeking Mino-Pimatisiwin: An Aboriginal Approach to Helping*. Halifax, Canada: Fernwood Publishing.

Healy, K. (1998) "Participation and child protection: The importance of context," *British Journal of Social Work*, 28: 897–914.

—— and Meagher, G. (2004) "The reprofessionalisation of social work: Collaborative approaches to achieving professional recognition," *British Journal of Social Work*, 34(2), 243–60.

—— and —— (2007) "Social workers' preparation for child protection: Revisiting the question of specialisation", *Australian Social Work*, 60(3): 321–35.

Heffernan, K. (2005) "Social work, New Public Management and the language of 'service user'," *British Journal of Social Work*, 36: 139–47.

Hendrick, H. (2003) *Child Welfare: Historical Dimensions, Contemporary Debate*, Bristol: Policy Press.

Hessle, S. (2000) "Child welfare on the eve of the twenty first century: What we have learned," in M. Callahan, S. Hessle and S. Strega (eds) *Valuing the Field: Child Welfare in an International Context*, Hampshire: Ashgate.

Hetherington, R., Cooper, A., Smith, P. and Wilford, G. (1997) *Protecting Children: Messages from Europe*, Lyme Regis: Russell House Publishing.

Hickman, D. (2003) "The role of fathers in the care and protection of children," *National Child Protection Clearinghouse Newsletter*, 11(1), Winter.

Higgins, D., Bromfield, L., Higgins, J. and Richardson, N. (2006) "Protecting Indigenous Children: Views of carers and young people on 'out-of-home care'," *Family Matters*, 75: 42–9.

Higgins, J., Bromfield, L. and Richardson, N. (2007) *Voices of Aboriginal and Torres Strait Islander Children and Young People in Care*, Issue Paper 7, Melbourne:

National Child Protection Clearinghouse, Australian Institute of Family Studies. Online. Available www.aifs.gov.au/nch/pubs/reports/promisingpractices/summary papers/menu.html (accessed November 9, 2007).

Hill, A. (2000) "A First Nations experience in First Nations child welfare services," in M. Callahan, S. Hessle and S. Strega (eds) *Valuing the Field: Child Welfare in an International Context*, Aldershot: Ashgate.

Hill, M. (1990) "The manifest and latent lessons of child abuse inquiries," *British Journal of Social Work*, 20: 197–213.

——, Stafford, A. and Lister-Green, P. (2002) "International Perspectives on Child Protection", Appendix B of Scottish Executive *It's Everyone's Job to Make Sure I'm Alright: Report of the Child Protection Audit and Review*, Edinburgh: Scottish Executive.

—— and Tisdall, K. (1997) *Children & Society*, Edinburgh: Pearson Education.

Hinman, L. (2003) *Ethics: A Pluralist Approach to Moral Theory*, Belmont, CA: Thomson Wadsworth.

Hirsch, P. and De Soucey, M. (2006) "Organizational restructuring and its consequences: Rhetorical and structural," *Annual Review of Sociology*, 32: 171–89.

HM Government (2005) *Every Child Matters: Change for Children*, London: Stationery Office.

Hodgkin, R. and Newell, P. (1998) *Implementation Handbook for the Convention on the Rights of the Child*, New York, Geneva, UNICEF.

Hojer, I. (2007) "Sons and daughters of foster carers and the impact of fostering on their everyday life," *Child and Family Social Work*, 12: 73–83.

Holland, S. (2000) "The assessment relationship: Interactions between social workers and parents in Child Protection Assessments," *British Journal of Social Work*, 30: 149–63.

—— and Scourfield, J. (2004) "Liberty and respect in child protection," *British Journal of Social Work*, 34(1): 21–36.

Holman, B. (1993) *A New Deal for Social Welfare: A Powerful Analysis of the Contract Culture*, London: Lion Books.

Holman, R. (1996) "Fifty years ago: The Curtis and Clyde reports," *Children & Society*, 10(3): 197–209.

Home Office, Department of Health, Department of Education and Science, and the Welsh Office (1991) *Working Together Under the Children Act 1989: A Guide to Arrangements for Inter-agency Co-operation for the Protection of Children from Abuse*, London: HMSO.

Hood, C., Rothstein, H. and Baldwin, R. (2001) *The Government of Risk: Understanding Risk Regulation Regimes*, Oxford: Oxford University Press.

Hornberger, S. and Briar-Lawson, K. (2005) "Advancing 21st-century child welfare through community building," *Child Welfare*, 84(2): 101–4.

Houston, S. and Griffiths, H. (2000) "Reflections on risk in child protection: is it time for a shift in paradigms?" *Child and Family Social Work*, 3: 1–10.

Hoyano, L. and Keenan, C. (2007) *Child Abuse: Law and Policy Across Boundaries*, Oxford: Oxford University Press.

Howe, D. (1992) "Child abuse and the bureaucratisation of social work," *Sociological Review*, 40(3): 491–508.

—— (1994) "Modernity, postmodernity and social work," *British Journal of Social Work*, 24(5): 513–32.

—— (1996) "Surface and Depth in Social Work Practice," in N. Parton (ed.) *Social Theory, Social Change and Social Work*, London: Routledge.

HREOC (1997) *Bringing them Home—Report of the National Inquiry into the Separation of Aboriginal and Torres Strait Islander Children from Their Families*, Canberra, ACT: Commonwealth of Australia.

Hudson, B. (2003) *Justice in the Risk Society*, London: Sage Publications.

Hugman, R. (2005) New Approaches in Ethics for the Caring Professions, London: Palgrave—Macmillan.

Humphreys, C. (2007) *Domestic Violence and Child Protection: Challenging Directions for Practice*, Sydney: Australian Domestic and Family Violence Clearing House.

Hutchinson, J. and Sudia, C. (2002) *Failed Child Welfare Policy: Family Preservation and the Orphaning of Child Welfare*, Lanham: University Press of America.

Hutchison, E. (1993) "Mandatory reporting laws: Child protection case findings gone awry," *Social Work*, 38: 56–62.

Igraham, F. and Matson, D. (1944) "Subdural hematoma in infancy", *Pediatrics*, 24: 1–37.

International Movement ATD Fourth World (2004) *"Valuing Children, Valuing Parents"; Focus on family in the fight against child poverty in Europe*, Pierrelaye, France: International Movement ATD Fourth World. Online. Available www.atd-fourthworld.org/Valuing-children-valuing-parents.html (accessed October 30, 2007).

Irwin, J., Waugh, F. and Bonner, M. (2006) "The inclusion of children and young people in research on domestic violence," *Communities, Children and Families Australia*, 1(1): 17–23.

Jack, G. (2004) "Child protection at the community level," *Child Abuse Review*, 13: 368–83.

Jenkins, P. (1998) *Moral Panic: Changing Concepts of the Child Molester in Modern America*, New Haven: Yale University Press.

Jenks, C. (1996) *Childhood*, London: Routledge.

Johnson, C., Sutton, E.S. and Thompson, D.M. (2005) "Child Welfare Reform in Minnesota," *Protecting Children*, 20(2 and 3): 55–61.

Johnson, S. and Petrie, S. (2004), "Child protection and risk-management: The death of Victoria Climbié," *Journal of Social Policy*, 33(2): 179–202.

Johnston, P. (1983) *Native children and the child welfare system*, Toronto: James Lorimor and Company.

Jones, A. and May, J. (1992) *Working in human service organisations: A critical introduction*, Melbourne: Longman Cheshire.

Jones, C. (2001) "Voices from the FrontLine: State social workers and New Labour," *British Journal of Social Work*, 31: 547–62.

Jones, H. and Davis, J. (1957) "Multiple traumatic lesions of the infant skeleton," *Stanford Medical Bulletin*, 15: 259–73.

Jordan, B. (2006) *Social Policy in the Twenty-First Century: New Perspectives, Big Issues*, Cambridge: Polity.

—— (2007) *Social Work and Well-being*, Lyme Regis: Russell House.

Kakabadse, A. (1982) *Cultures of the Social Services*, Aldershot: Gower.

Kamerman, S. and Kahn, A. (1990) "If CPS is driving child welfare—where do we go from here?" *Public Welfare*, 48 (Winter): 9–13.

Kapp, S. and Vella, R. (2004) "The unheard client: Assessing the satisfaction of parents of children in foster care," *Child and Family Social Work*, 9: 197–206.

Kempe, H., Silverman, F., Steele, B., Droegemueller, W. and Silver, H. (1962) "The battered child syndrome," *Journal of the American Medical Association*, 181: 17–24.

Kemshall, H. (2002) *Risk, Social Policy and Welfare*, Buckingham: Open University Press.

Khoo, E.G., Hyvönen, U. and Nygren, I. (2002) "Child welfare protection: Uncovering Swedish and Canadian orientations to social intervention in child maltreatment," *Qualitative Social Work*, 1(4): 451–71.

Kirkpatrick, I., Ackroyd, S. and Walker, R. (2005) *The New Managerialism and Public Service Professions*. Basingstoke: Palgrave Macmillan.

Kotter, J. (2007) "Leading change—Why transformation efforts fail," *Harvard Business Review*, 85(1): 96–103.

Laming Report (2003) *The Victoria Climbié Inquiry: Report of the Inquiry by Lord Laming* (Cm 5730), London: The Stationery Office.

Lawrence, A. (2004) *Principles of Child Protection: Management and Practice*, Berkshire, England: Open University Press.

Leeson, C. (2007) "My life in care: experiences of non-participation in decision-making processes," *Child and Family Social Work*, 12: 268–77.

Leschied, A.W., Chiodo, D., Whitehead, P.C., Hurley, D. & Marshall, L. (2003) "The empirical basis of risk assessment in child welfare: The accuracy of risk assessment and clinical judgment," *Child Welfare*, 82(5): 527–40.

Levitas, R. (1998) *The Inclusive Society: Social Exclusion and New Labor*, Basingstoke: Macmillan.

Lewis, O., Sargent, J., Chaffin, M., Friedrich, W., Cunningham, N., Cantor, P., Coffey, P., Villani, S., Beard, P., Clifft, M. A. and Greenspun, D. (2004) "Progress Report on the Development of Child Abuse Prevention, Identification, and Treatment Systems in Eastern Europe," *Child Abuse and Neglect*, 28: 93–111.

Lipsky, M. (1980) *Street-level Bureaucracy: Dilemmas of the Individual in Public Services*, New York: Russell Sage Foundation.

Littlechild, B. (2005) "The nature and effects of violence against child-protection social workers: Providing effective support," *British Journal of Social Work*, 35: 387–401.

Loman, A.L. and Siegel, G.L. (2005) "Alternative response in Minnesota: Findings of the program evaluation," *Protecting Children*, 20(2–3): 79–92.

Lombardi, J. (2003) *Time To Care. Redesigning Child Care to Promote Education, Support Families, and Build Communities*, Philadelphia: Temple University Press.

London Borough of Brent (1985) *A Child in Trust: Report of the Panel of Inquiry Investigating the Circumstances Surrounding the Death of Jasmine Beckford*, London: London Borough of Brent.

London Borough of Greenwich (1987) *A Child in Mind: Protection in a Responsible Society; Report of the Commission of Inquiry into the Circumstances Surrounding the Death of Kimberley Carlile*, London: London Borough of Greenwich.

London Borough of Lambeth (1987) *Whose Child? The Report of the Panel Appointed to Inquire into the Death of Tyra Henry*, London: London Borough of Lambeth.

Lonne, B. (2003) "Social Workers and Human Service Practitioners," in M. Dollard, A.Winefield and H. Winefield (eds) *Occupational Stress in the Service Professions*, London: Taylor & Francis.

—— and Cheers, B. (2004a) "Retaining rural workers: An Australian study," *Rural Society*, 14(2), 163–77.

—— and —— (2004b) "Practitioners speak: A balanced account of rural practice, recruitment and retention," *Rural Social Work*, 9: 244–54.

——, McDonald, C. and Fox, T. (2004) "Ethical Practice in the Contemporary Human Services," *Journal of Social Work*, 4(3): 345–67.

—— and Thomson, J. (2005) "Critical review of Queensland's Crime and Misconduct Commission Inquiry into abuse of children in foster care: Social work's contribution to reform," *Australian Social Work*, 58(1): 86–99.

Love, C. (2006) "Maori perspectives on collaboration and colonisation in contemporary Aotearoa/New Zealand child and family welfare policies and practices," in N. Freymond and G. Cameron (eds) *Toward Positive Systems of Child and Family Welfare: International Comparisons of Child Protection, Family Service, and Community Caring Systems*, Toronto: University of Toronto Press.

McAuliffe, D. (2005) "I'm still standing: Impacts and consequences of ethical dilemmas for social workers in direct practice," *Journal of Social Work Values and Ethics*, 2: 1–10.

McBeath, G. and Webb, S. (2002) "Virtue ethics and social work: Being lucky, realistic and not doing one's duty", *British Journal of Social Work*, 32: 1015–36.

McCallum, S. and Eades, D. (2001) "Response to *New Directions* in child protection and family support in Western Australia: a policy initiative to re-focus child welfare practice," *Child and Family Social Work*, 6(3): 269–74.

McConnell, D. and Llewellyn, G. (2005) "Social inequality, 'the deviant parent' and child protection practice," *Australian Journal of Social Issues*, 40(4): 553–66.

McDonald, C. (2006) *Challenging Social Work: The Context of Practice*, Basingstoke, Hampshire: Palgrave Macmillan.

——, Harris, J. and Wintersteen, R. (2003) "Contingent on context? Social work and the state in Australia, Britain, and the USA," *British Journal of Social Work*, 33(2): 191–208.

MacDonald, G. (1990) "Allocating blame in social work," *British Journal of Social Work*, 20: 545–6.

MacIntyre, A. (1981) *After Virtue: A Study in Moral Theory*, London: Duckworth.

Maclay, F., Bunce, M. and Purves, D. (2006) "Surviving the system as a foster carer," *Adoption and Fostering*, 30(1): 29–38.

McLean, J. and Andrew, T. (2000) "Commitment, satisfaction, stress and control among social services managers and social workers in the UK," *Administration in Social Work*, 23(4): 93–117.

Mallon, G. and McCartt, P. (eds) (2005) *Child Welfare for the 21st Century: A Handbook of Practices, Policies and Programs*, New York: Columbia University Press.

Maluccio, A., Ainsworth, F. and Thoburn, J. (2000) *Child Welfare Outcome Research in the United States, the United Kingdom and Australia*, Washington DC: CWLA Press.

Mansell, J. (2006a) "Stabilisation of the statutory child protection response: Managing to a specified level of risk assurance," *Social Policy Journal of New Zealand*, 28: 77–96.

—— (2006b) "The underlying instability in statutory child protection: Understanding the system dynamics driving risk assurance levels," *Social Policy Journal of New Zealand*, 28: 97–132.

Mason, J. and Gibson, C. (2004) *The Needs of Children in Care—A report on a research project: Developing a model of out-of-home care to meet the needs of individual children, through participatory research which includes children and young people*, Sydney: Social Justice and Social Change Research Center, University of Western Sydney and Social Justice and Research Program, Uniting Care Burnside.

Mathews, B. and Kenny, M. (2008) "Mandatory Reporting Legislation in the United States, Canada, and Australia: A Cross-Jurisdictional Review of Key Features, Differences, and Issues," *Child Maltreatment*, 13: 50–63.

Meagher, G. and Healy, K. (2006) *Who cares? Volume 2: Employment structure and incomes in the Australian care workforce*, Strawberry Hills, NSW, Australia: Australian Council of Social Service.

—— and Parton, N. (2004) "Modernising social work and the ethics of care," *Social Work & Society*, 2(1),10–27.

Melton, G. (1993) "Is There A Place For Children In The New World Order?," *Notre Dame Journal of Law, Ethics, and Public Policy, 7*, 491–532.

—— (2002) "Chronic Neglect of Family Violence: More than a Decade of Reports to Guide U. S. Policy," *Child Abuse and Neglect*, 26: 569–86.

—— (2005) "Mandated reporting: a policy without reason," *Child Abuse and Neglect*, 25(1): 9–18.

Melton, G. and Holaday, B. (eds) (2008) "Strong Communities as Safe Havens for Children" [Special issue], *Family and Community Health*, 13(2).

—— and Thompson, R. (2002) "The conceptual foundation: Why child protection should be neighborhood-based and child-centered," in G. Melton, R. Thompson and M. Small (eds) *Toward a Child-centered, Neighborhood-based Child Protection System: A report on the consortium on children, families and the law*, Westport, Connecticut: Praeger.

——, —— and Small, M. (2002) (eds) *Toward a Child-centered, Neighborhood-based Child Protection System: A report on the consortium on children, families and the law*, Westport, CT: Praeger.

Mendes, P. (2005) "Graduating from the child welfare system: A case study of the leaving care debate in Victoria Australia," *Journal of Social Work*, 5(2): 155–71.

—— and Moslehuddin, B. (2004) "Graduating from the Child Welfare System: A Comparison of the UK and Australian Leaving Care Debates," *International Journal of Social Welfare*, 13: 332–9.

Merrick, D. (2006) *Social Work and Child Abuse: Still Walking the Tightrope?* 2nd edn, London: Routledge.

Meuller, F. and Carter, C. (2005) "The 'HRM project' and managerialism: Or why some discourses are more equal than others," *Journal of Organizational Change*, 18(4): 369–82.

Meyer, M. and Zucker, L. (1989) *Permanently Failing Organizations*, Newbury Park, CA: Sage Publications.

Mildred, J. (2003) "Claimsmakers in the child sexual abuse 'wars': Who are they and what do they want?" *Social Work*, 48(4): 492–503.

Miller, D. (1959) "Fractures among children: Parental assault as causative agent," *Minnesota Medicine*, 42: 1209–13.

Milner, J. (1993) "A disappearing act: The differing career paths of fathers and mothers in child protection investigations", *Critical Social Policy*, 38: 48–63.

Mitchell, L., Barth, R., Green, R., Wall, A., Biemer, P., Berrick, J. and Webb, M. (2005) "Child welfare reform in the United States: Findings from a local agency survey," *Child Welfare*, 84(1): 5–24.

Monckton, Sir W. (1945) *Report on the Circumstances which led to the Boarding-Out of Dennis and Terence O'Neil at Bank Farm, and the Steps Taken to Supervise their Welfare* (Cmd 6636), London: HMSO.

Mor Barak, M.E., Nissly, J.A. and Levin, A. (2001) "Antecedents to retention and turnover among child welfare, social work, and other human service employees: What can we learn from past research? A review and meta-analysis," *The Social Service Review*, 75 (4): 625–61.

Morgan, R. (2007) *Children and Safeguarding: Children's Views for the DfES Priority Review*, Commission for Social Care Inspection, London, January. Online. Available www.csci.gov.uk/PDF/children_and_safeguarding.pdf (accessed December 5, 2007).

Morris, J. (2005) "For the children: Accounting for careers in child protective services," *Journal of Sociology & Social Welfare*, 32(2): 131–45.

Mudaly, N. and Goddard, C. (2006) *The Truth is Longer than a Lie: Children's Experiences of Abuse and Professional Interventions*, London: Jessica Kingsley.

Munro, E. (1999a) "Common errors of reasoning in child protection work," *Child Abuse & Neglect*, 23(8): 745–58.

—— (1999b) "Protecting children in an anxious society," *Health, Risk & Society*, 1(1): 117–27.

—— (2002) *Effective Child Protection*, London: Sage.

—— (2004a) "The impact of audit on social work," *British Journal of Social Work*, 34: 1075–95.

—— (2004b) "The impact of child abuse inquiries since 1980," in N. Stanley and J. Manthorpe (eds) *The Age of Inquiry: Learning and Blaming in Health and Social Care*, London: Routledge.

—— and Parton, N. (2007) "How far is England in the process of introducing a Mandatory Reporting System?" *Child Abuse Review*, 16(1): 5–16.

Myers, J. (1994) (ed.) *The Backlash: Child Protection Under Fire*, Thousand Oaks, CA: Sage.

National Inquiry into the Separation of Aboriginal and Torres Strait Islander Children from their Families (1997), *Bringing Them Home*, Canberra, Australia: Australian Government Printing Service.

Neff, R. (2004) "Achieving justice in child protection," *Journal of Sociology and Social Welfare*, 31(1): 137–54.

Nelson, B. (1984) *Making an Issue of Child Abuse and Neglect: Political Agenda Setting for Social Problems*, Chicago: University of Chicago Press.

Neu, D. and Therrien, R. (2003) *Accounting for Genocide: Canada's Bureaucratic Assault on Aboriginal People*, New York: Zed Books.

Neuberger, J. (2005) *The Moral State We're In: A Manifesto for 21st Century Society*, London: Harper Collins Publishers.

Niebuhr, H. (1963) *The Responsible Self: An Essay in Christian Moral Philosophy*, New York: Harper & Row.

NSPCC Inform (2004) *Child Protection Statistics—Child Protection in the Community*. Online. Available https://www.nspcc.org.uk/Inform/resourcesforprofessionals/Statistics/CPStats/community_wdf48755.pdf (accessed November 30, 2007).

Nunno, M. (2006) "Invited Commentary—The effects of ARC organizational intervention on caseworker turnover, climate, and culture in children's services systems," *Child Abuse and Neglect*, 30: 849–54.

Nutt, L. (2006) *The Lives of Foster Carers: Private Sacrifices, Public Restrictions*, London: Routledge.

Oakley, J. and Cocking, D. (2001) *Virtue Ethics and Professional Roles*, Cambridge: Cambridge University Press.

Office of the United Nations High Commissioner for Human Rights (2007) *Legislative History of the Convention on the Rights of the Child* (Vol. 2), New York and Geneva: United Nations.

Osborn, A. and Delfabbro, P. (2006) "An analysis of the social background and placement history of children with multiple complex needs in Australian out-of-home care," *Communities, Children and Families Australia*, 1(1): 33–42.

Packman, J. (1981) *The Child's Generation*, 2nd edn, Oxford: Basil Blackwell and Martin Robertson.

Parker, R. (1995) "A Brief History of Child Protection," in E. Farmer and M. Owen (eds) *Child Protection Practice: Private Risks and Public Remedies*, London: HMSO.

Parton, N. (1985) *The Politics of Child Abuse*, Basingstoke: Macmillan.

—— (1991) *Governing the Family: Child Care, Child Protection and the State*, Basingstoke: Macmillan.

—— (1996) "Social work, risk and 'the blaming system'," in N. Parton (ed.) *Social Theory, Social Change and Social Work*, London: Routledge.

—— (ed.) (1997) *Child Protection and Family Support: Tensions, Contradictions and Possibilities*, London: Routledge.

—— (2006a) *Safeguarding Childhood: Early Intervention and Surveillance in a Late Modern Society*, Basingstoke: Palgrave/Macmillan.

—— (2006b) "'Every Child Matters': The shift to prevention while strengthening protection in children's services in England," *Children and Youth Services Review*, 28(8): 976–92.

—— (2007) "Changes in the Form of Knowledge in Social Work: From the 'social' to the 'informational'?" *British Journal of Social Work*. Online. Available http://bjsw.oxfordjournals.org.ezproxy.library.uq.edu.au/cgi/reprint/bcl337v1 (accessed March 30, 2007).

—— (2008) "The 'Change for Children' programme in England: Toward the preventive-surveillance state," *Journal of Law and Society*, 35(1): 166–87.

—— and Mathews, R. (2001) "New directions in child protection and family support in Western Australia: a policy initiative to re-focus child welfare practice," *Child and Family Social Work*, 6(2): 97–113.

—— and O'Byrne, P. (2000) *Constructive Social Work: Toward a New Practice*, Basingstoke: Palgrave.

——, Thorpe, D. and Wattam, C. (1997) *Child Protection: Risk and the Moral Order*, Basingstoke: Macmillan.

Pecora, P., Kessler R., O'Brien K., Williams J., Hirpie, E. and Morello, S. (2003) *Assessing the Effects of Foster Care: Early Results from the Casey National Alumni Study*. Seattle, WA: Casey Family Programs. Online. Available www. casey.org/Resources/Publications/NationalAlumniStudy.htm (Accessed November 30, 2007).

——, ——, Williams, J., O'Brien, K., Downs, C., English, D., White, J., Hiripi, E., White, C., Wiggins, T. and Holmes, K. (2005) *Improving Family Foster Care: Findings from the Northwest Foster Care Alumni Study*, Seattle, WA: Casey Family Programs. Online. Available www.casey.org/Resources/Publications/Northwest AlumniStudy.htm (accessed November 30, 2007).

——, Williams, J., Kessler, R., Hiripi, E., O'Brien, K., Emerson, J., Herrick, M. and Torres, D. (2006) "Assessing the educational achievements of adults who were formerly placed in family foster care," *Child and Family Social Work*, 11: 220–31.

——, Whittaker, J., Maluccio, A. and Barth, R. (eds) (2007) *The Child Welfare Challenge: Policy, Practice and Research*, 2nd edn, New Jersey: Transaction Publishers.

Pelton, L.H. (2008) "Informing child welfare: The promise and limits of empirical research", in D. Lindsey and A. Schlonsky (eds) *Child Welfare Research*, New York: Oxford University Press.

Penglase, J. (2005) *Orphans of the Living: Growing up in Care in Twentieth Century Australia*, Fremantle, Western Australia: Curtin University Press.

Pennell, J. (2004) "Family group conferencing in child welfare; Responsive and regulatory interfaces," *Journal of Sociology and Social Welfare*, 31(1): 117–35.

Pharr, S. and Putnam, R. (eds) (2000) *Disaffected Democracies: What's Troubling the Trilateral Countries*, Princeton, NJ: Princeton University Press.

Pinkerton, J. (2002) "Child Protection," in R. Adams, L. Dominelli and M. Payne (eds) *Critical Practice in Social Work*, Basingstoke, Hampshire: Palgrave MacMillan.

Pittman, J.F. and Buckley, R.R. (2006) "Comparing maltreating fathers and mothers in terms of personal distress, interpersonal functioning, and perceptions of family climate," *Child Abuse and Neglect*, 30: 481–96.

Power, M. (1994) "The Audit Society," in A.G. Hopwood and P. Miller (eds) *Accounting as Social and Institutional Practice*, Cambridge: Cambridge University Press.

—— (1997) *The Audit Society: Rituals of Verification*, Oxford: Oxford University Press.

Prilleltensky, I. and Prilleltensky, O. (2006) *Promoting Well-Being. Linking Personal, Organizational and Community Change*, New Jersey: John Wiley & Sons.

Pringle, K. (1998) *Children and social welfare in Europe*, Buckingham: Open University Press.

Proulx, J. and Perrault, S. (2000) *No Place for Violence: Canadian Aboriginal Alternatives*, Nova Scotia, Canada: Fernwood Publishing and RESOLVE.

Putnam, R. (2000) *Bowling Alone: The Collapse and Revival of American Community*, New York: Simon & Schuster.

Read, J., Mosher, L. and Bentall, R. (2004) *Models of Madness*, New York: Routledge.

Reder, P., Duncan, S. and Gray, M. (1993) *Beyond Blame: Child Abuse Tragedies Revisited*, London: Routledge.

Reed, C. (1999) "Managerialism and social welfare: A challenge to public administration", *Public Administration Review*, 59(3): 263–6.

Regehr, C., Hemsworth, D., Leslie, B., Howe, P., and Chau, S. (2004) "Predictors of post-traumatic distress in child welfare workers: A linear structural equation model," *Child and Youth Services Review*, 26: 331–46.

Reich, J. (2005) *Fixing Families: Parents. Power and the Child Welfare System*, New York: Routledge.

Roberts, D. (2002) *Shattered Bonds: The Color of Child Welfare*, New York: Basic Civitas Books.

Rose, W. (1994) "An overview of the development of services—the relationship between protection and family support and the intentions of the Children Act 1989," *Department of Health Paper for Sieff Conference*, September 5, Cumberland Lodge.

Ross, R. (1992) *Dancing with a Ghost: Exploring Indian Reality*, Markham Ontario: Octopus Publishing Group.

Ruch, G. (2005) "Relationship based practice and reflective practice: Holistic approaches to contemporary child care social work," *Child and Family Social Work*, 10: 111–23.

Rustin, M. (2004) "Learning from the Victoria Climbié Inquiry," *Journal of Social Work Practice*, 18(1): 9–18.

SafeCare Inc. (2007) *SafeCare's Philosophy*. Online. Available www.safecare.com.au/us/philosophy.htm (accessed October 14, 2007).

Savicki, V. (2002) *Burnout across Thirteen Cultures: Stress and Coping in Child and Youth Care Workers*, London: Praeger.

Sawyer, R. and Lohrbach, S. (2005) "Differential response in child protection: Selecting a pathway," *Protecting Children*, 20(2 and 3): 44–54.

Schorr, L. (1998) *Common Purpose: Strengthening Families and Neighborhoods to Rebuild America*, New York: Anchor Books.

Scott, D. (2006a) "Sowing the seeds of innovation in child protection," keynote presentation at the *10th Australasian Child Abuse and Neglect Conference*, Wellington, New Zealand.

—— (2006b) "Toward a public health model of child protection in Australia," *Communities, Children and Families Australia*, 1(1): 9–16.

—— and O'Neil, D. (1996) *Beyond Child Rescue*, Australia: Allen & Unwin.

—— and Swain, S. (2002) *Confronting Cruelty: Historical Perspectives on Child Protection in Australia*, Melbourne: Melbourne University Press.

Scott, E. (2006) "From family crisis to state crisis: The impact of overload on child protection in New South Wales," paper presented at *Children in a Changing World—Getting it Right*, 16th ISPCAN International Congress on Child Abuse and Neglect, York.

Scottish Executive (2005) *An Inspection into the Care and Protection of Children in Eilean Siar*, Edinburgh: Scottish Executive.

Scourfield, J. (2003) *Gender and Child Protection*, Basingstoke: Palgrave Macmillan.

—— (2006) "The challenge of engaging fathers in the child protection process," *Critical Social Policy*, 26(2): 440–9.

—— and Welsh, I. (2003) "Risk, reflexivity and social control in child protection: New times or same old story?" *Critical Social Policy*, 23(3): 398–420.

Secretary of State for Social Services (1974) *Report of the Inquiry into the Care and Supervision Provided in Relation to Maria Colwell*, London: HMSO.

—— (1988) *Report of the Inquiry into Child Abuse in Cleveland* (Cm 412), London: HMSO.

Sennett, R. (2003) *Respect: The Formation of Character in an Age of Inequality*, London: Penguin Books.

Shireman, J. (2003) *Critical Issues in Child Welfare*, New York: Columbia University Press.

Shlonsky, A. and Wagner, D. (2005) "The next step: Integrating actuarial risk assessment and clinical judgement into an evidence-based practice framework in CPS case management," *Children and Youth Services Review*, 27: 409–27.

Shook Slack, K., Holl, J., Lee, B., McDaniel, M., Altenbernd, L. and Stevens, A. (2003) "Child protective intervention in the context of welfare reform: The effects of work and welfare on maltreatment reports," *Journal of Policy Analysis and Management*, 22(4): 517–36.

Shusterman, G.R., Fluke, J.D., Hollinshead, D.M. and Yuun, Y.Y.T. (2005) "Alternative responses to child maltreatment: Findings from NCANDS," *Protecting Children*, 20(2 and 3): 32–43.

Silverman, F. (1953) "The Roentgen manifestations of unrecognized skeletal trauma in infants," *American Journal of Roentgenology, Radium Therapy and Nuclear Medicine*, 69: 413–27.

Sinclair, T. (2000) "Destructive Discourses: Child Protection and Systematically Distorted Communication," paper presented at *Sociological Sites/Sights*, TASA Conference, Adelaide: Flinders University.

Small, M., Melton, G., Olson, K. and Tomkins, A. (2002) "Creating caring communities: The need for structural change," in G. Melton, R. Thompson and M. Small (eds) *Toward a Child-Centered Neighborhood-Based Child Protection System: A Report on the Consortium on Children, Families and the Law*, Westport, Connecticut: Praeger.

Smith, A. (1944) "The beaten child," *Hygeia*, 22: 386–8.

Smith, B. (2005) "Job retention in child welfare: Effects of perceived organizational support, supervisor support, and intrinsic job value," *Children and Youth Services Review*, 27: 153–69.

Smith, C. (2001) "Trust and confidence: Possibilities for social work in high modernity," *British Journal of Social Work*, 31(2): 287–305.

Smith, D. and Donovan, S. (2003) "Child welfare practice in organizational and institutional context," *Social Service Review*, 77(4): 541–63.

Smith, M., Nursten, J. and McMahon, L. (2004) "Social workers' responses to experiences of fear," *British Journal of Social Work*, 34: 541–59.

Smith, R. (2005) *Values and Practices in Children's Services*, Hampshire: Palgrave Macmillan.

Spears, W. and Cross, M. (2003) "How do 'children who foster' perceive fostering?" *Adoption and Fostering*, 27(4): 38–45.

Spratt, T. and Callan, J. (2004) "Parents' views on social work interventions in child welfare cases," *British Journal of Social Work*, 34(2): 199–224.

Stalker, K. (2003) "Managing risk and uncertainty in social work," *Journal of Social Work*, 3(2): 211–33.

Stanley, J. and Goddard, C. (2002) *In the Firing Line: Violence and Power in Child Protection Work*, Chichester: John Wiley and Sons.

Stanley, N. and Manthorpe, J. (2004) *The Age of the Inquiry: Learning and Blaming in Health and Social Care*, New York: Routledge.

——, Penhale, B., Riordan, D., Barbour, S. and Holden, S. (2003) *Child Protection and Mental Health Services*, Bristol: The Policy Press.

Statham, J. and Aldgate, J. (2003) "From legislation to practice: Learning from the Children Act 1989 Research Program," *Children & Society*, 17(2): 149–56.

Stein, M. (2006) "Research review: Young people leaving care," *Child & Family Social Work*, 11: 273–9.

Stevens, M. and Higgins, D. (2002) "The influence of risk and protective factors on burnout experienced by those who work with maltreated children," *Child Abuse Review*, 11: 313–31.

Stewart-Weeks, M. (2000) "Trick or Treat: social capital, leadership and the new public policy," in I. Winter (ed.) *Social Capital and Public Policy in Australia*, Melbourne: Australian Institute of Family Studies.

Stoez, D. (2007) "Can child protective services be reformed?" in H. Karger, J. Midgley, P. Kindle and C. Brown (eds) *Controversial Issues in Social Policy*, 3rd edn, Boston: Pearson.

Sunday Mail (2007) "System failed my son: Mum—Tragic life of bashed tot," October 7, 2007 p.4. Online. Available www.news.com.au/couriermail/story/0,23739,22542820-3102,00.html (accessed October 9, 2007).

Swift, K.J. (1997) "Canada: Trends and issues in child welfare," in N. Gilbert (ed.) *Combating Child Abuse: International Perspectives and Trends*, Oxford: Oxford University Press.

Testro, P. and Peltola, C. (2007) *Rethinking Child Protection: A New Paradigm?—A discussion paper*, Brisbane, Australia: Peak Care Queensland Inc.

Tew, J. (2006) "Understanding power and powerlessness: Toward a framework for emancipatory practice in social work," *Journal of Social Work*, 6(1): 33–51.

Thoburn, J., Wilding, J. and Watson, J. (2000) *Family Support in Cases of Emotional Maltreatment and Neglect*, London: Stationery Office.

Thomas, N. (2002) *Children, Family and the State: Decision-making and child protection*, Bristol: The Policy Press.

Thompson, I., Melia, K, and Boyd, K. (2000) *Nursing Ethics*, 4th edn, Edinburgh: Churchill Livingstone.

Thompson, N., Stradling, S., Murphy, M. and O'Neill, P. (1996) "Stress and organizational culture," *British Journal of Social Work*, 26: 647–65.

Thomson, J. (2007) "Child protection workers' perceptions of foster care and foster carers: A study in Queensland," *Australian Social Work*, 60(3): 336–46.

—— and Thorpe, R. (2004) "Powerful partnerships in social work: group work with parents of children in care," *Australian Social Work*, 57(1): 46–56.

Thorpe, D. (1994) *Evaluating Child Protection*, Buckingham: Open University Press.

—— (1997) "Policing minority child rearing practices in Australia: the consistency of 'child abuse',"in N. Parton (ed.) *Child Protection and Family Support: Tensions, Contradictions and Possibilities*, London: Routledge.

Thorpe, R. (2007) "Building Bridges in Working with (not against) Families," Keynote paper presented at *Borders and Bridges, National Conference of the Australian College of Child Protection and Family Practitioners*, Melbourne, May.

—— and Westerhuis, D. (2006) "You need to walk in their shoes: Foster carers' views on what makes a good foster carer," paper presented at the *Working Together for Families, CROCCS 4th International Conference, Sydney*, 4–6 August.

Tilbury, C. (2004) "The influence of performance measurement on child welfare policy and practice," *British Journal of Social Work*, 34(2): 225–41.

—— (2005) "Child protection services in Queensland post-Forde Inquiry," *Children Australia*, 30(3): 10–16.

—— (2006) "Accountability via performance measurement: The case of child protection services," *Australian Journal of Public Administration*, 65(3): 48–61.

Tobin, B. (1994) "Codes of Ethics: Why we also need practical wisdom," *Australian Psychiatry*, 2(2): 55–7.

Tomison, A. (2004) *Current Issues in Child Protection Policy and Practice: Informing the NT Department of Health and Community Services Child Protection Review*, Melbourne: National Child Protection Clearing House, Australian Institute of Family Studies.

Toqueville, A. de (S. Kessler ed.; S. Grant trans.) (2000) *Democracy in America*, Indianapolis: Hackett (Originally published 1835).

Trocme, N., Tam, K.K. and McPhee, D. (1995) "Correlates of substantiation of maltreatment in child welfare investigations," in J. Hudson and B. Galaway (eds) *Child Welfare in Canada: Research and Policy Implications*, Toronto: Thomson Educational Publishing.

Tronto, J. (1993) *Moral Boundaries: A Political Argument for an Ethic of Care*, New York: Routledge.

Trotter, C. (2004) *Helping Abused Children and their Families: Toward an Evidence-based Practice Model*, Sydney: Allen and Unwin.

TSA (2007) *New policies for lighters, electronics and breast milk*, Washington, DC: TSA. Online. Available www.tsa.gov/travellers/sop/index.shtm (accessed October 26, 2007).

Tsui, M. and Cheung, F. (2004) "Gone with the wind: The impacts of managerialism on human services," *British Journal of Social Work*, 34: 437–42.

Tunstill, J. and Aldgate, J. (2000) *Services for Children in Need: From Policy to Practice*, London: Stationery Office.

Turnell, A. and Edwards, S. (1999) *Signs of Safety: A Solution and Safety Oriented Approach to Child Protection Casework*, New York: W. Norton & Co.

UN (1989) *Convention on the Rights of the Child*, UN Doc. A/Res/44/25.

Urek, M. (2005) "Making a case in social work: The construction of an unsuitable mother," *Qualitative Social Work*, 4(4): 451–67.

US Advisory Board on Child Abuse and Neglect (1990) *Child Abuse and Neglect: Critical First Steps in Response to a National Emergency*, Washington, DC: US Government Printing Office.

—— (1991) *Creating Caring Communities: Blueprint for an Effective Federal Policy on Child Abuse and Neglect*, Washington, DC: US Government Printing Office.

—— (1993) *Neighbors Helping Neighbors: A New National Strategy for the Protection of Children*, Washington, DC: US Government Printing Office.

US Department of Health and Human Services (1993) *Neighbours Helping Neighbours: A New National Strategy for the Protection of Children*, Washington DC: US Government Printing Office.

—— (2001) *National Study of Child Protective Services Systems and Reform Efforts: Literature Review*. Online. Available http://gov/cps-status03 (accessed September 6, 2006).

—— (2003) *National Study of Child Protective Services Systems and Reform Efforts: Review of State CPS Policy*. Online. Available http://aspe.hhs.gov/cps-status03 (accessed September 6, 2006).

Victorian Government Department of Human Services (2007) *Every Child every Chance: A Good Childhood is in Everyone's Interests—Cumulative Harm: An Overview*, Best interests series, Melbourne: Victorian Government Department of Human Services.

Wade, J. and Dixon, J. (2006) "Making a home, finding a job: Investigating early housing and employment outcomes for young people leaving care," *Child and Family Social Work*, 11: 199–208.

Waldfogel, J. (1998) *The Future of Child Protection: How to Break the Cycle of Abuse and Neglect*, Cambridge, MA: Harvard University Press.

—— (2008) "The future of child protection revisited," in D. Lindsey and A. Schlonsky (eds) *Child Welfare Research*, New York: Oxford University Press.

Walter, J. (2006) "Ministers, minders and public servants: Changing parameters of responsibility in Australia," *Australian Journal of Public Administration*, 65(3): 22–7.

Warner, J. (2003) "An initial assessment of the extent to which risk factors, frequently identified in research, are taken into account when assessing risk in child protection cases," *Journal of Social Work*, 3(3): 339–63.

Watson, J. (2004) *Child Neglect Literature Review*, Ashfield, NSW: Center for Planning & Research.

Watson, S. and Moran, A. (2005) (eds) *Trust, Risk and Uncertainty*, Hampshire: Palgrave Macmillan.

Wattam, C. (2002) "Making Enquiries under Section 47 of the Children Act 1989," in K. Wilson and A. James (eds) *The Child Protection Handbook*, 2nd edn, London: Balliere Tindall.

Weaver, D., Chang, J., Clark, S. and Rhee, S. (2007) "Keeping public child welfare workers on the job," *Administration in Social Work*, 31(2): 5–25.

Webb, S. (2006) *Social Work in a Risk Society: Social and Political Perspectives*, Hampshire: Palgrave Macmillan.

Weber, Z. (2006) "Professional values and ethical practice," in A. O'Hara and Z. Weber (eds) *Skills for Human Service Practice*, Melbourne: Oxford University Press.

Wells, R. (2006) "Managing child welfare agencies: What do we know about what works?" *Children and Youth Services Review*, 28: 1181–94.

Westrum, R. (2004) "A typology of organisational cultures", *Quality and Safety in Health Care*, 13(ii): 22–7.

Wharf, B. (2002) *Community Work Approaches to Child Welfare*, Peterborough: Broadview Press.

Whiting Blome, W. and Steib, S. (2004) "Whatever the problem, the answer is 'evidence-based practice'—Or is it?" *Child Welfare*, 83: 611–15.

Wilson, K., Sinclair, I. and Gibbs, I. (2000) "The trouble with foster care: The impact of stressful 'events' on foster carers," *British Journal of Social Work*, 30: 193–209.

——, Fyson, R. and Newstone, S. (2007) "Foster fathers: their experiences and contributions to fostering," *Child and Family Social Work*, 12: 22–31.

Wooley, H.P. and Evans Jr, W. (1955) "Significance of skeletal lesions in infants resembling those of traumatic origin," *Journal of American Medical Association*, 158: 539–43.

Zapf, M.K. (2004) "Concluding thoughts from social work," in N. Bala, M.K. Zapf, R. Williams, R. Vogel and J. Hornick (eds) *Canadian Child Welfare Law: Children, Families and the State*, Toronto: Thomson Educational Publishing.

——, Pelech, W., Bastien, B., Bodor, R., Carriere, J. and Zuk, G. (2003) "Promoting anti-oppressive social work education: the University of Calgary's access learning circle model," in W. Shera (ed.) *Emerging Perspectives on Anti-oppressive Practice*, Toronto: Canadian Scholar's Press.

Index